The Ab Revolution™

4th edition, expanded

Jolie Bookspan, MEd, PhD, FAWM

Stop Back Pain from Swayback
Healthier Daily Life
More Effective Exercise

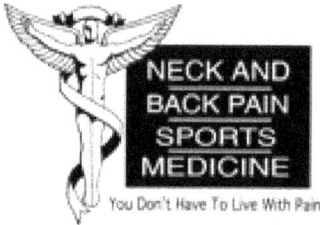

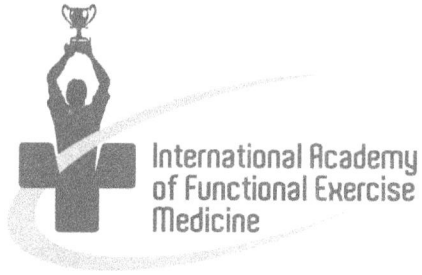

NECK AND
BACK PAIN
SPORTS
MEDICINE
You Don't Have To Live With Pain

International Academy
of Functional Exercise
Medicine

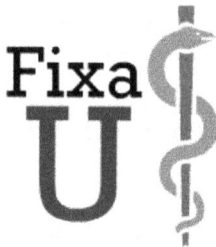

Fixa
U

http://drbookspan.com/

Dedication

To my grandmother, who showed me real exercise, body mechanics, and health from my earliest years. She got her college degree at age 81. To her the highest things in life were education and Jack LaLanne.

To my mother. I promised her when I was four years old that I would find how to end back pain.

To my students and patients, who all feel better and work their abs more using this method. They showed me how needed it is.

To my wonderful husband and hero, Paul. What beautiful abs you have, my dear.

Dear 4th Edition Readers

The Ab Revolution teaches how to fix a common slouch and the pain it causes, and get stronger healthier daily life and exercise for core and body.

This new 4th edition has additions to text, organization, and illustrations. Readers asked for both simple line drawings and photographs to better see concepts and application. Concepts are restated in several places, giving readers latitude to skip to desired topics. Most explanations previously introducing Parts I and II are moved to Part III so that you can learn healthy spine position to stop back pain right away in Part I, and learn healthier exercises one after the next in Part II. Then, Part III explains all about why.

If you have expertise to make a better edition through better electronic formatting, adding movies, or typo corrections, contact me. I will add them with credit to you. We can exchange expertise. Contact instructions are on the Projects page of my web site:
http://drbookspan.com/Projects.html

The front cover photograph of this book deliberately pokes good-natured fun of conventional "ab" advertising, featuring hyperlordotic (swayback) spine indicating lack of knowledge that abdominal muscles are supposed to prevent that.

Thank you for all the requests for more Ab Revolution. Go use your brains and abs to have fun with *The Ab Revolution*.

Table of Contents

Part I – Using The Ab Revolution to Stop Back Pain From Hyperlordosis

Part II – Using The Ab Revolution for Better Core and Whole Body Strengthening and Stretching

Part III – Understanding Abs and The Ab Revolution

Introduction
Dedication   iii
Dear 4th Edition Readers   iv
Table of Contents   v
Foreword by Andrew Seigel, Third Degree Black Belt   ix
What Is The Ab Revolution™?   x

Part I Using the Ab Revolution™ for Back Pain Control   1
Key Points Part I   1
What Kind of Back Pain Can The Ab Revolution Help?   2
Does The Ab Revolution Hurt?   4
How Do I Know If I Am Doing It Right?   4
What Does Hyperlordosis / Swayback Look Like?   5
A Few Ways to Fix Hyperlordosis and Learn Neutral Spine   10
Visualize How Abs Work to Reduce Lower Back Pain   20
Ab Exercises And Core Strengthening Don't Automatically
Change Posture, Lumbar Angle, or Lower Back Pain   22
Prevent Back Pain From Hyperlordosis, Walking and Running   24
Prevent Back Pain In Heeled Shoes, and "Tip-Toe"   27
How to Prevent Lower Back Pain When Reaching Overhead   29
How to Prevent Lower Back Pain When Carrying Loads in Front   32
Prevent Lower Back Pain from Hyperlordosis During Pregnancy   34
Prevent Lower Back Pain When Carrying Loads On Your Back   35
Shoulder Bags And Babies Carried On The Hip   37
Prevent Back Pain From Hyperlordosis, Swimming and SCUBA   38

How To Stop Back Pain From Hyperlordosis From Golf   40
When Your Lower Back Hurts to Lie Flat Without A Pillow   41
A Little About Disc Injury and Flexion   46
Disc Injury and Hyperlordosis   49
Can Someone With Herniated Discs, Osteoporosis, Upper
Crossed Syndrome, Hernia Use The Ab Revolution?   50
Stop Back Pain When Sitting - Not Rounded, Not Arched   52
Get Up from Sitting   54
Reference Sheet For Healthy Bending, Reaching, and Lifting   55

**Part II Ab Revolution™ Exercises for Healthier, More Effective,
Core and Whole Body Strengthening and Stretching   56**
Key Points Part II   56
What Is Different About Ab Revolution Exercises?   57
How to Use Ab Revolution for Squats   58
How to Use Ab Revolution When Lifting Overhead   60
Putting Squat and Lift Together in One Continuous Exercise   61
Using Ab Revolution To Fix Triceps Curls   62
Using Ab Revolution To Fix Lunges   63
Special Ab Revolution Exercise – Isometric Abs   64
Why Isn't It Necessary To Keep Knees Bent?   66
Ab Revolution Neutral Spine Planks   68
Ab Revolution Planks Lifting Arms and Legs   71
Ab Revolution Pushups With Neutral Spine   73
Ab Revolution Plank Rows   75
Ab Revolution High Planks With Neutral Spine - Handstand   76
High Plank or Wall Handstand With Rows   77
Walking And Jumping Pushups (Spiders)   81
The Flag   82
Using Oblique Abs to Control Spine—Side Arm Planks   83
Benefit to Wrists   84
More Challenging Moves for Oblique Abdominal Muscles   85
Use Abs, Not Hands, to Reposition the Spine For Leg Lifts   86
Back Leg Lifts   88
Using Ab Revolution for Chin-ups and Pull-ups   91
Using Ab Revolution for Pull-Downs   92
Using Ab Revolution for Handstands and Headstands   93

Ab Revolution Bands and Cables   94
Ab Revolution Bands and Cables for Oblique Training   95
Ab Revolution Bands and Cables for Training Throwing and
Other Overhead Arm Activities for Sports   97
Medicine Ball, Kettlebell, India Club, And Heavy Objects   98
Knife and Other Target Throwing   99
Ab Revolution Neutral Spine For Archery and Target Sports   100
Ab Revolution Using an Exercise Ball   101
Ab Revolution Abdominal Twists   106
Ab Revolution for Punching   108
Ab Revolution Punching Using Bands Or Cables   111
Using Abdominal Muscles For Pushing   113
Ab Revolution for Kicking   114
Ab Revolution Using Bands to Train Kicking   115
Back Extension Without Compressive Hyperlordosis   116
Supported Extension For Headstands and Handstands   119
Ab Revolution For Stretching The Spine   120
Using Ab Revolution For Balancing Stretches Like Tree Pose   123
Ab Revolution For Stretching Arms Overhead   124
Ab Revolution For Stretching Quadriceps and Anterior Hip   126
Real Athletes Need Neutral Spine   128

Part III –Understanding Abs and The Ab Revolution   **129**
What Exactly Do Abs Do?   130
What Do Gluteal Muscles Do?   132
Using Abs Doesn't Mean Sucking In or Making Them Tight   134
Why Do People With Hyperlordotic Back Pain Often Feel
They Need To Bend Forward To Feel Better?   136
Is Hyperlordosis Natural?   137
Ab Revolution Exercises Work Your Abs the Way You Need
For Real Life - Functional Exercise   138
Problems of Hyperlordosis During Exercise   139
When Does Hyperlordosis Occur?   141
Difference Between Lordosis, Hyperlordosis, and Swayback?   142
What About Ab Rocking Devices?   143
What About Ab Machines?   144
What About Ab Isolators?   146
What About Electronic Ab Zapper Belts?   147
What About Miracle Liquids and Fat Burners?   148

What About Neoprene Waist Bands?   149
How Do You Flatten Your Abdomen?   150
How Do You Get "Washboard Abs?"   151
How Many, How Often?   152
"Ab-Only" Exercises Are Not Functional   153
What About "The Ab Study?"   154
What's Wrong with Crunches?   155
What Are All the Muscles Called?   157
Will Ab Revolution Exercises Hurt The Neck Or Back?   160
Should You Work Your Abs Every Day or Every Other Day?   161
Is The Ab Revolution Researched As Effective?   162
Why Is This Method Called a Revolution?   164
What Instructors and Trainers Say About The Ab Revolution   167
What Black Belt Martial Artists Say About The Ab Revolution 168
What Medical Doctors Say About The Ab Revolution   169
More Resources   171
Credits   173
About the Author   174

Foreword by Andrew Seigel, Third Degree Black Belt

I bought this book after attending a seminar with this extraordinary lady—more on that in a moment. This book is invaluable to anyone who wants to eliminate back-pain immediately. Most of us have been told so many times to "stand up straight, don't slouch" that we do precisely the wrong thing: leaning back, over-arching and putting strain and stress on our back each and every day. With Dr. Bookspan's straightforward, no-nonsense approach, you can instantly modify a key bad posture and the pain/ache in your lower back IS GONE. What is deceptive is how easy this is to accomplish and so on first read, you might not totally grasp the concept. Take your time with the book, try each modification and exercise as she clearly explains it, and give it a try. Your first goal should be to stop the pain, your second to start strengthening your abs and back by retraining your daily habits - and let me tell you, you'll thank her for it.

As a 40-year-old martial arts instructor with 24 years experience, I was fortunate enough to attend one of her seminars. That's where she really works her magic, face to face. She utilized the concepts in her book to change the way a room full of martial arts instructors and grandmasters live their daily lives. For all of our knowledge and experience, Dr. Bookspan provided a collective epiphany to over 60 veteran martial artists, we were all shaking our heads in amazement and smiling at how good our backs felt. It's practical and it works. To her credit, Dr. Bookspan lives her healthy lifestyle philosophy. This book is not very big, nor is Dr. Bookspan, but both are filled with tremendous power and wisdom. Everyone could benefit from The Ab Revolution.

What Is The Ab Revolution™?

A change in understanding and use of abdominal muscles

The Ab Revolution teaches you how to stop hyperlordosis, a slouch that is a major cause of one kind of back pain. Changing hyperlordosis to neutral spine is quick to learn. Then you use the new neutral spine position for all you do. The Ab Revolution has two parts:

Part I shows how to stop one kind of lower back pain from too much inward curve in the lower spine called swayback, hyperlordosis, overarch, and other terms. Hyperlordosis pain is usually felt from standing, walking, overhead reaching, running, and other times when you slouch into swayback posture. Part I teaches how to reposition your spine from painful swayback to healthy pain-free angle. Done correctly, lower back pain from hyperlordosis stops right then without exercises, strengthening, or "tightening." After that, you maintain healthy vertebral angle during daily life so that you no longer have the cause of the pain. It is not exercises that stop back pain, but stopping the painful swayback. Neutral spine uses your abdominal muscles, giving you healthful, built-in core use from the new healthier way you stand and move for all you do.

Part II shows you how to use neutral spine for innovative exercise from simple to the toughest you can get. You learn healthier, more effective core exercise, plus healthier exercise for your body as a whole. More than stand-alone exercises to "do" a number of repetitions then stop, these are retraining drills to train and practice neutral spine. These Ab Revolution exercises can be done in the gym, weight room, at home, and for sports. You can choose a variety of the drills to use together with music for a high-energy fitness class.

Part III gives science and explanations. In previous editions, many of these long sections were in Part I to introduce and expand concepts, and in Part II to explain better exercise. This 4th edition moves most of them to Part III so you may begin using this method more quickly and simply.

The Ab Revolution, as a whole, teaches you to change spine angle from hyperlordosis to neutral during standing, walking, running, sitting, ordinary daily activities, and a large variety of exercise. This is a large difference in understanding and using "abs" instead of doing "sets and reps" of conventional flexion exercises. The Ab Revolution, as a whole, teaches you to use abdominal and core muscles the way you need them in real life.

Part I
Using The Ab Revolution™ for Back Pain Control

Key Points Part I

A common kind of back pain occurs from too much inward lumbar curve, called hyperlordosis or swayback of the lumbar spine. The Ab Revolution is a direct way to stop that unhealthy posture to stop that source of back pain during all you do.

No exercises or weeks of strengthening are needed to stop hyperlordosis and back pain from it. You move your lumbar spine from swayed to neutral, as quickly and easily as moving any other part of your body. Once you learn neutral spine, you use it to prevent back pain during all your ordinary daily movement.

Part I starts with teaching how to change hyperlordosis to neutral spine. All the rest of Part I shows using it for all your normal daily activities. Functional core use goes on all day using healthy spine position for all you do.

Understanding the overall concept is more important and useful than spending time on tiny details.

The Ab Revolution does not hurt. If you get pain, you are doing it wrong. Stop and see if you are moving as intended, or skip and check what other causes of pain you may have.

After you learn to stop hyperlordosis and use neutral spine in Part I, if you want to learn healthier exercise using it, see Part II.

What Kind of Back Pain Can The Ab Revolution Help?

The Ab Revolution method was developed to stop back pain from hyperlordosis also called swayback, including S.I. syndrome (sacroiliac) and facet pain. By moving spine position to stop hyperlordosis (swayback), you can quickly stop the pain that results. No exercises do this. You move your spine to healthier position, the same as moving your arm or leg when and where wanted. The Ab Revolution teaches you how.

Spondylolisthesis occurs when one lower vertebra slips forward or backward on the next, adding to increased inward lumbar curve and hyperlordosis. In an ongoing cycle, increasing hyperlordosis worsens spondylolisthesis. Using The Ab Revolution for healthful position during daily activities and exercise, reduces the painfully increased vertebral angle, to reduce, even stop, pain and deformity.

Hyperlordosis reduces needed space around spinal nerves and discs, increasing pain from existing conditions such as stenosis (narrowed spine areas) and impingement (things being pressed upon). In spinal stenosis, bending forward is often prescribed for pain relief to enlarge the constricted posterior space, leading to patients bent over walkers, or walking around bent over, which is not healthy for the spine or body over the long run. Using the increased posterior spacing of neutral spine instead, provides healthier pain relief in many cases, while standing upright.

Someone with reduced lumbar lordosis (flat back) may be helped by Ab Revolution repositioning. Reduced spine flexibility has less tolerance for slouching to end range. Even a small slouch may pressure a less mobile spine. Other people diagnosed with "flat back" may sway the spine from a higher segment, causing pain from hyperlordosis higher up. Another consideration is that someone with pronounced hyperlordosis may be misdiagnosed as "flat back" when they overly lean backwards, which gives a misleading flatter appearance. For those who flatten the lumbar area from rounding their lumbar spine forward (slouching forward), learning a more neutral angle is designed to restore healthier, pain-free position.

The habit of bending over forward to lift objects (instead of good bending with upright torso and "using the legs"), and years of using forward-bending exercises and stretches, is a large contributor to degenerating and herniated discs. Disc injury is only briefly addressed in this book. To stop disc pain and damage, you need to stop that separate cause. The Ab Revolution method is not a primary fix for disc pain, but if someone with disc pain and sciatica also slouches in a way that increases lower back curve in a way that increases their pain, this will take away pain from that component. Occasionally, discs or other damaged structures may protrude in directions that make neutral spine uncomfortable. Don't force neutral. Stopping main causes of disc injury still needs addressing. Some resources for that are listed at the end of Part III.

This method includes healthy squatting, which is healthy bending. Using good neutral spine bending for all the things you need to retrieve and lift from the floor instead of disc-injuring bending over forward will prevent ongoing disc injury from habitual bad bending. Identifying and stopping hyperlordosis may also be useful for people who are misdiagnosed with disc pain. In many cases, bulging discs are asymptomatic, and in reality, some or all the pain comes from another source. Check with your health providers before using any of this method if you are unsure of causes.

If you do not slouch your lumbar spine in hyperlordosis, and already have neutral spine, and your pain is from something else, then this technique to learn and practice neutral spine would not change your cause of pain. Check causes of that pain and fix those causes. You can still use The Ab Revolution to get better exercise, shown in Part II, as long as you do not do them in any way hurts.

Does The Ab Revolution Hurt?

The purpose of The Ab Revolution is to identify and correct hyperlordosis, which is a painful spine position, and to use healthy pain-free position instead. When using The Ab Revolution, if you have pain, you ARE doing it wrong. Stop and see if you are moving as this method intends. Part I explains how.

When using Ab Revolution exercises in Part II, you should feel effort, work, exercise, stretch, but not back pain. Stop and assess. If you have other injuries that prevent healthy movement, check those causes and address them.

How Do You Know If You Are Doing It Right?

If you feel a distinct change to stopping lumbar pressure or pain when you tilt to neutral, and you feel abdominal muscles working more, then you know you are doing it right. You may feel pleasant stretch in the lower back. It should look better and feel better.

What Does Hyperlordosis / Swayback Look Like?

In hyperlordosis, the normal slight inward lumbar curve increases. The resulting sharper angle compresses and pinches the lower spine, making it ache. Three common slouches increase lumbar curve: anterior hip tilt, leaning the upper body backward (thoracic lean-back) and pushing the whole pelvis forward. People may combine some or all of these slouches. This section describes each. The section after this one gives several drills to learn to correct each.

Anterior Hip Tilt

With anterior hip tilt, the line down the side of the pelvis tilts forward. The belt line tips downward in front. (Right photo below.)

With neutral spine, belt line is horizontal, not tilted. The line down the side of the pelvis to the side of the upper leg bone (greater trochanter) is vertical (Left photo below.)

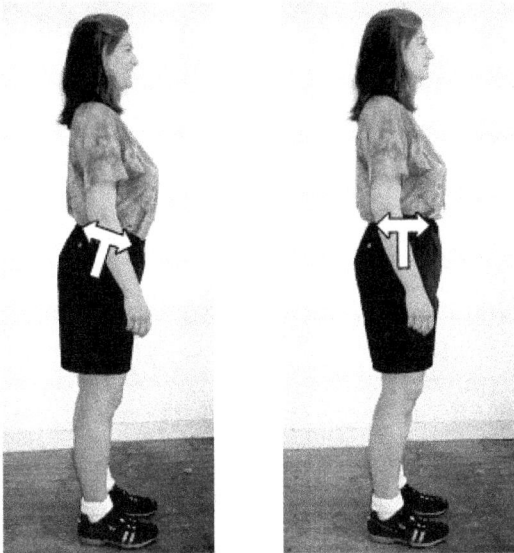

Left: Hyperlordosis from anterior tilt. Pelvis tilts forward. Belt line tilts downward in front. Hip tilts outward in back.
Right: Corrected to neutral by tucking the pelvis under until vertical. Belt line becomes level.

Leaning The Upper Body Backwards - Thoracic Lean-Back

Leaning the upper body backward increases lower spine inward angle. The folded area compresses the lower spine under the weight of the upper body.

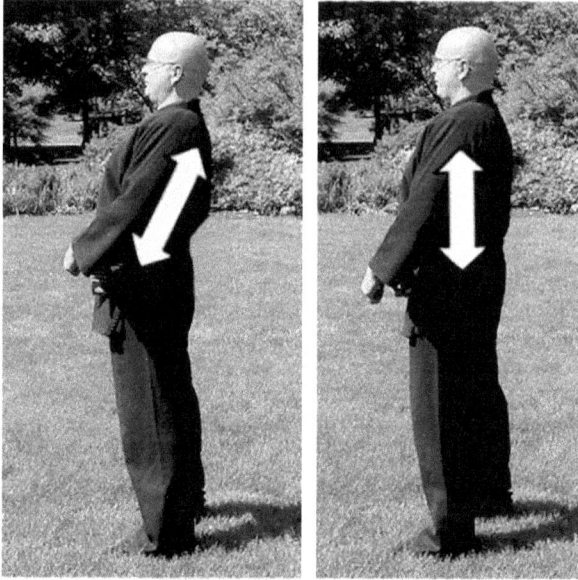

Left: Hyperlordosis from leaning the upper body backwards
Right: Neutral spine with upper body vertical.

With neutral spine, the upper body is vertical, not leaning backwards. To correct hyperlordosis from a thoracic lean-back, bring the upper body forward to upright vertical position. The movement is of the upper body as a whole without rounding the shoulders, or using the shoulders at all. No movement is needed from the hip, unless there is separate slouch component.

Relation to Upper Back Pain. The common suggestion to "bring shoulders back" to correct "round-shoulder" posture often results in leaning backward, increasing hyperlordosis. Instead of "bringing shoulders back" to correct rounded upper body, straighten and "unround" the upper spine. It is the upper spine, not shoulders, that needs straightening.

Hip Pushed Forward

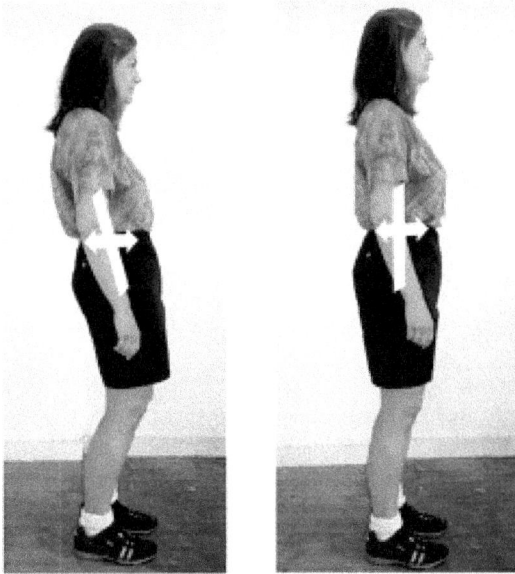

Left: Entire pelvis is pushed forward.
Right: Corrected to neutral spine and vertical.

Pushing the pelvis forward is not the same as the "hip tuck" movement that changes pelvic angle to vertical. Pushing forward makes hyperlordosis greater, not less.

Some people push the pelvis forward thinking it is a hip tuck, and wonder why their hyperlordosis pain does not go away. Other think they are "bringing shoulders back," and instead, lean the entire upper body backwards and push the pelvis forward.

A "pelvis forward" hyperlordosis is corrected by bringing the entire pelvis back until the body as a whole is vertical. Straighten the upper spine ("unround" the upper back) until upright.

Anterior Hip Tilt and Thoracic Lean-Back Combined

Some people do both anterior hip tilt and thoracic lean:

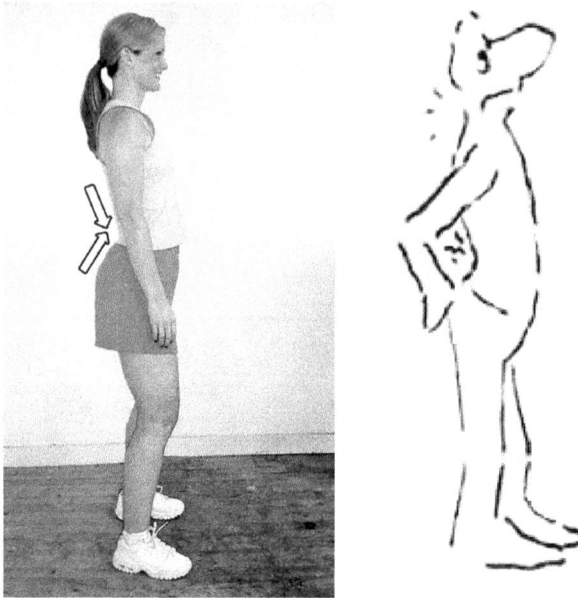

Anterior hip tilt (pelvis tips forward, belt line downward in front) plus thoracic lean (upper body leans backward).

To stop the pain from hyperlordosis with two causes, you need to correct both components. Correct the anterior hip by "tucking the hip" from tilted to vertical, and correct the thoracic lean-back by bringing the upper body forward to upright and straight. Do not be fooled by the common posture rule of "keep the shoulder over the hip." As you can see from the photograph and drawing above, the shoulder is aligned over the hip, but the problem lies between the two.

Simple Lines Show Kinds Of Hyperlordosis

The drawing below shows, from left to right, #1 neutral spine with vertical pelvis and thorax, #2 anterior hip tilt, #3 upper body (thoracic) lean-back #4 pelvis pushed forward.

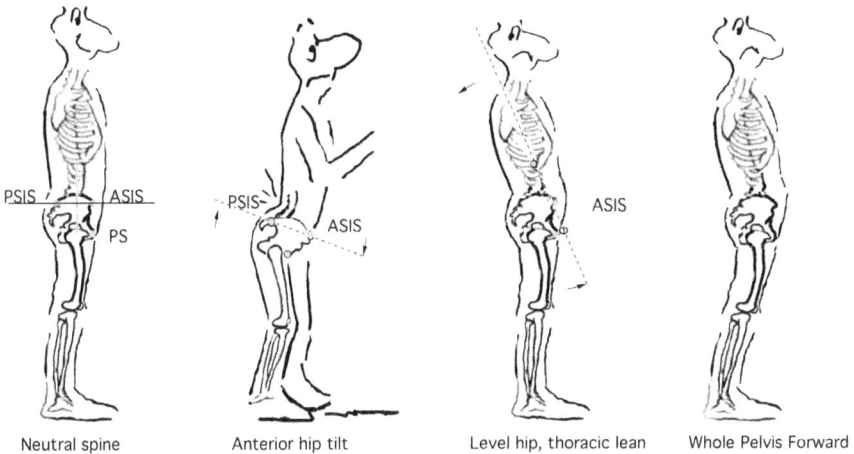

Neutral spine   Anterior hip tilt   Level hip, thoracic lean   Whole Pelvis Forward

Neutral Spine: Belt line, or the line from the back of your pelvic bone top bump (medical abbreviation PSIS) to the top bump in front (ASIS) is approximately horizontal. The line down the side of the hip to the upper leg is vertical. Sight inward lumbar curve remains.

Anterior Hip Tilt: Belt line tips downward in front—the line from the top bump in the back of the pelvis (PSIS) to top bump in front (ASIS). The line down the side of the hip to the leg, like a stripe or seam on the side of clothing, tilts forward. So does the line from the ASIS to the pelvic bones in front, called the symphysis pubis (PS).

Upper Body Lean-Back (Thoracic Lean-Back): The upper body leans backward. The hip may be level. Very commonly mistaken for "standing up straight."

Pelvis Pushed Forward: The entire pelvis pushes forward. Sometimes mistaken for flat back, but it increases hyperlordosis.

A Few Ways to Fix Hyperlordosis and Learn Neutral Spine

This section shows a few ways to learn neutral spine. They are all different ways to learn the same thing—reducing a large lower spine curve to a healthy small pain-free one. Some people have trouble envisioning or feeling the change using one way, but find another easier or clearer. Try each until one, or hopefully all, make sense and you can easily move your spine out of hyperlordosis into neutral.

All of the examples are intended to work right away to show you how to make a simple position change. A common assumption is that abdominal exercise to strengthen abdominal muscles will change posture or stop back pain. Strengthening does not do either automatically. Even exercises called posture exercises do not fix posture. To change posture, you move your body. Like using arm muscles to move your arm, you use abdominal muscles to move your spine to healthy position right then.

Many people cannot imagine using abdominal muscles when standing to control posture. They only know about tightening or lying down to do forward bending abdominal exercises in fitness classes. It is irony, as those are not healthful, or the way you move in real life.

For all the methods, remember, all movement to change swayback to neutral comes from the spine. There is no tightening of any muscles. There is no "sucking in" and no "navel to spine." That is not how you move in real life and does not work to learn or use neutral spine.

Neutral spine does not mean rigid, stiff, fixed position. Health does not come from lack of movement. Don't do anything that hurts. Used as intended, you should feel better right then. If not, stop, re-read, understand first, then fix it.

Learn to Fix Hyperlordosis Method 1 - Push Your Lower Back Against a Wall

This is often the easiest for most people. If this looks understandable, start here, relax, and use all you learn with this drill to do the others until it all becomes clear and natural:

1. Stand with your back against a wall. Touch your backside and upper back to the wall. For now, don't worry about head position.

2. Notice the space between your lower back and the wall. Press that space closer toward the wall. Feel the hip change tilt. Don't let your upper back round or move forward from the wall. Relax your abdomen and breathe normally.

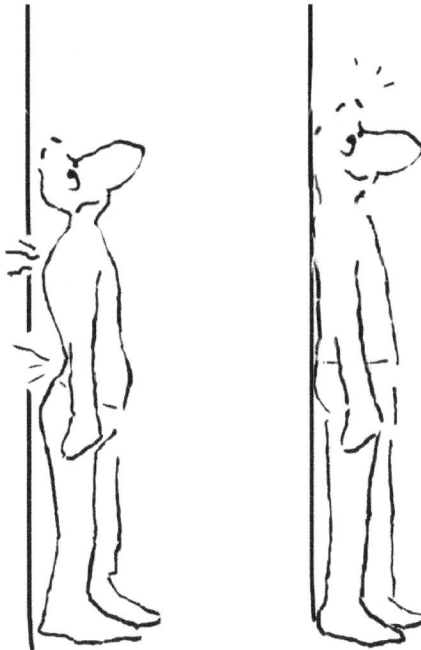

Left: Hyperlordosis. Large lumbar sway. Belt line downward (anterior pelvic tilt), Upper body leans backward (thoracic lean).
Right: Lower back closer to wall. Beltline level. Torso upright. Small neutral lumbar curve.

Some people benefit by putting one hand in the space between their lower back and the wall and pressing their lower back against their hand. They can better tell what their lower back is doing.

Notice how it feels like a slight crunch standing up, but you do not round your upper body away from the wall or slouch the upper body. Your pelvis rotates (tucks) under until it no longer tilts outward in back, but is vertical.

Do not tighten anything. Don't tighten your abdominals in front, or gluteal (backside) muscles in back. Learn how to move without tightening. Just as you can't tighten your legs and run well, tightening (clenching, pressing, bracing, locking, pressing, splinting) muscles restricts healthy movement and life. Learn to move without tightening.

When walking or running, if you feel the familiar swayback causing back pain, and can't remember how to correct it, you can find a wall or tree to test and correct positioning.

Wall Push With Arms Overhead
Once you understand how to reduce lumbar sway by reducing lumbar distance from a wall, stay at the wall and lift both arms by your head so that your fingers touch the wall.

Notice if you increase lower back curve to raise arms. Press your lower back toward the wall. Correct spine positioning to neutral.

Notice if you can't raise your arms as high with neutral spine. This is valuable information. It can mean that you have been causing or increasing hyperlordosis each time you reach. It may also indicate you don't have the shoulder range you think you have.

If needed, use the *anterior stretches*, described later in Part I, starting with, "When Your Lower Back Hurts to Lie Flat Without A Pillow."

Fix Hyperlordosis Method 2 - Visual With Hands

1. Stand with one hand at the top of your ribs and the other on your front pelvic bones (hands at top and bottom of your abs). Feel and see how far apart you hands are. Use a mirror to help.

2. Move your spine so that your hands come closer together. The movement is like a small crunch while standing. Feel your spine moving. Feel that you reduce hyperlordosis (too large inward lumbar curve) to a smaller curve. You may feel a pleasant stretch.

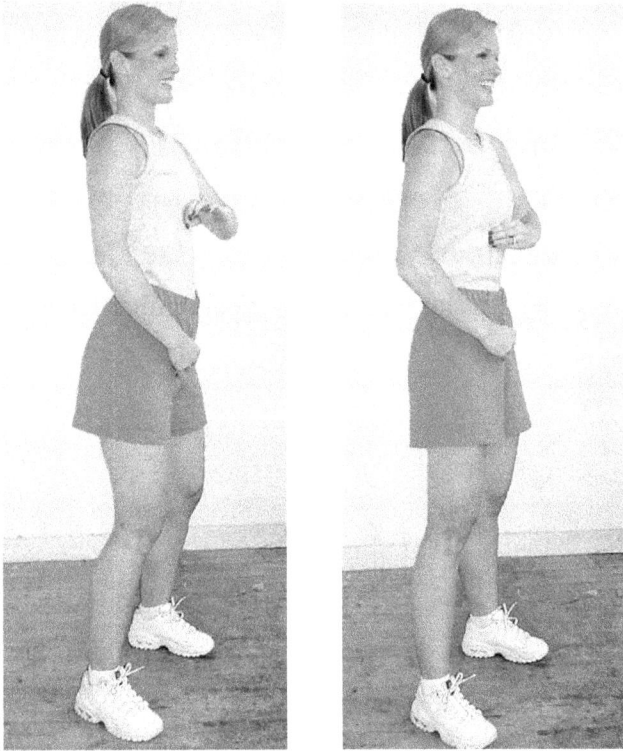

Left: Hyperlordosis. Beltline tilts downward (anterior pelvis tilt). Upper body leans backward, (thoracic lean-back), ribs are up in front. Right: Bringing abdominal muscles to shorter length to bring ribs down to level and pelvis straightened to vertical. Neutral spine is produced. Level belt line. Vertical torso.

Pull only enough to change leaning back to upright and vertical without rounding the upper body. Tuck the hip to change angle from tilted forward to vertical, with belt line horizontal.

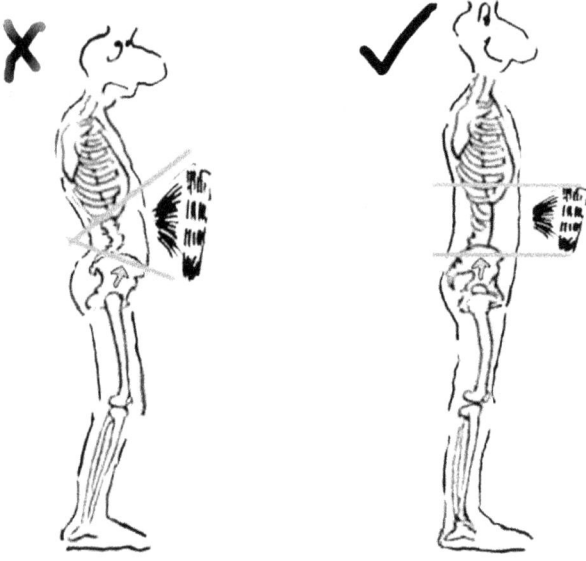

Feel abdominal length shorten in front. Feel lumbar length lengthen in back.

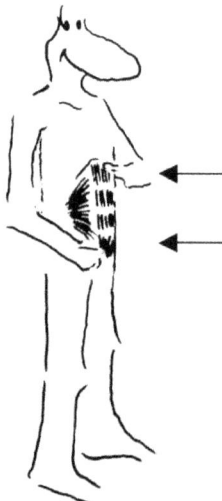

Distance between your hands roughly represents abdominal muscle length.

Fix Hyperlordosis Method 3 - Thumbs

1. Stand with hands on hips, thumbs to the back and fingers over the front of the hipbone.

2. Tilt your pelvis under so that your thumbs come downward in back. Use the same spine movement of a small standing crunch, as in each of the previously shown methods.

3. Don't push the pelvis forward. Only change the tilt.

4. Once you are in neutral spine, remember to relax your abdomen to breathe normally. Feel and practice how you can change the tilt of the pelvis using abdominal muscles without tightening or restricting breathing.

Users have reported that this method helps them to remember and feel the tilt change during walking and running.

A short video of this method is on my web site summary article: http://drbookspan.com/AbsArticle

Fix Hyperlordosis Method 4 - Standing Crunch

This drill uses a partial abdominal crunch while standing upright.

1. Stand and make a tucking or flexing motion with your torso, as if doing a small crunch while standing.

2. Feel your ribs pull downward and forward. Feel the bottom of your hip swing under.

3. Do this only enough to stand upright and straight, not curled forward. A slight inward curve remains in the lower back.

Some people like to think of a full bucket that needs to be held level.

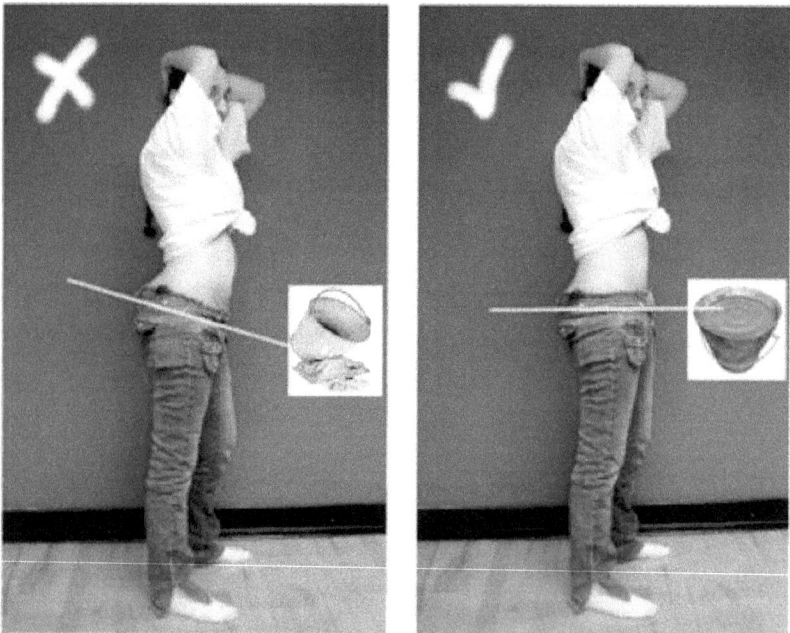

Left: Hyperlordosis. Large lumbar sway. Beltline tilts downward (anterior pelvic tilt) Upper body leans backward, (thoracic lean). Rib line tips upward. Right: Neutral spine. Level belt line. Upright torso.

Fix Hyperlordosis Method 5 - Hands and Knees

This drill can help people who can't figure out neutral spine when standing. This drill is also useful for learning neutral spine planks and pushups, and other hand-supported drills in Part II.

1. Go to a "hands and knees" position. Notice if you sag your lower spine downward (or try it for this drill), shown below.

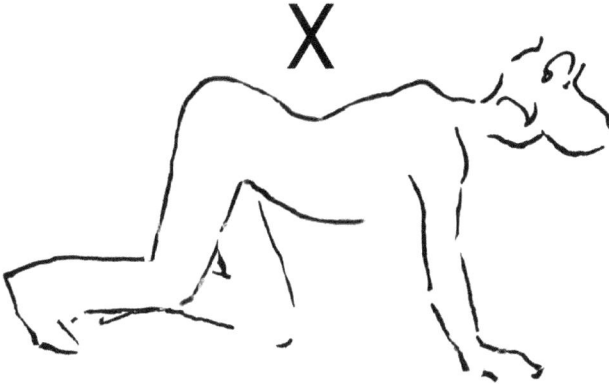

2. Tuck the backside under, and lift the lower back, until the spine straightens and the back is flat, as in the drawing below.

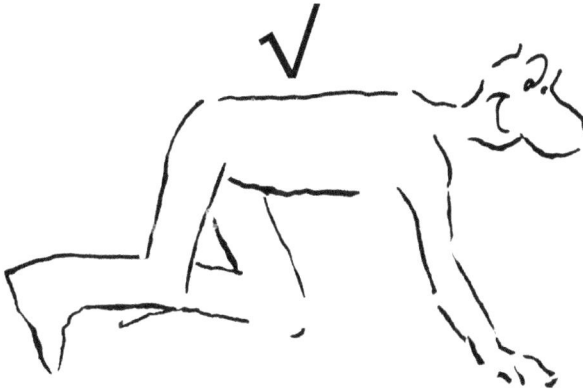

Changing sagging spine to neutral is not an exercise to do 10 times. Ideally, you only need it once, to learn needed spine movement. Once you learn how to change swayback to neutral, use the new neutral position when you stand up and for all else you do.

Fix Hyperlordosis Method 6 - Floor Push (Floor Pelvic Tilt)

1. Lie on your back with straight legs. Notice if your lower spine arches upward off the floor, or try it for this drill, but not if it makes pain.

2. Press your lower back toward the floor. Feel and learn the motion needed. Keep legs straight on the floor.

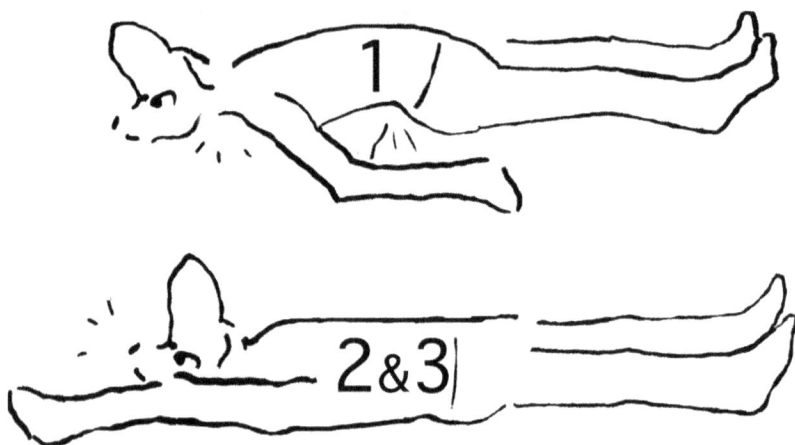

3. Once you can control lumbar arch lying flat, practice neutral spine with arms overhead, for learning how to stand and reach overhead with neutral spine.

Lying on the floor and reducing lumbar arch by tilting the pelvis is often used in physical therapy as a "pelvic tilt." It is often misunderstood, and thought of as a strengthener. It is given as an exercise to do a number of times without understanding that doing a number of tilts is not what helps the back.

Tilts are not nearly enough to strengthen anything. Even if they could, strengthening does not change a hyperlordotic posture. Doing tilts does not teach how to use it to reduce hyperlordosis to neutral spine when you actually need it—when standing. Use this drill to learn the movement. Ideally you only need to try it a few times lying down to understand what to do the rest of the time when standing.

Watch Other People

Watch other people when they exercise, walk, run, reach, and go about their daily lives. Notice hyperlordosis. Examples are shown in the photos below. Use it as a helpful reminder to correct your own painful habits right then to healthy movement habits.

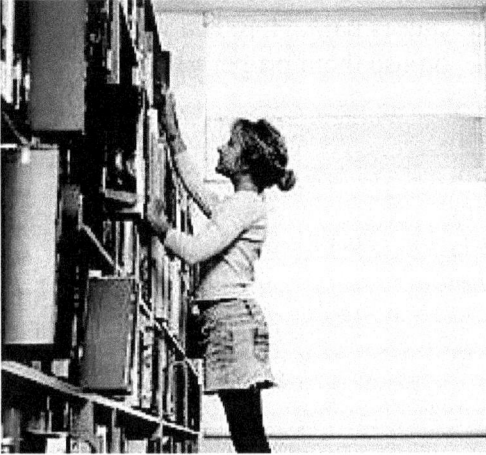

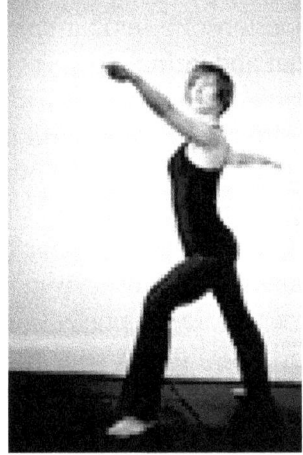

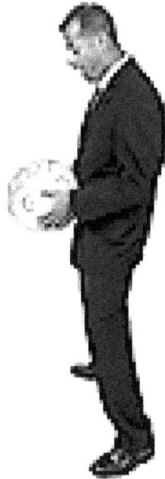

Visualize How Abs Work to Reduce Lower Back Pain

People usually have a vague idea that abdominal muscles have something to do with helping the back, but they don't know specifically what ab muscles do, or that they don't do it automatically. You may have the strongest abs and never use them to stop hyperlordotic lumbar spine that causes pain. Here is a way to visualize what abdominal muscles do, if you use them properly:

1. Hold your right hand up with thumb facing you. Your palm represents the front of your body. The back of your hand is your back. Curl your fingers forward to represent abs at work. Straighten your fingers to simulate using back muscles.

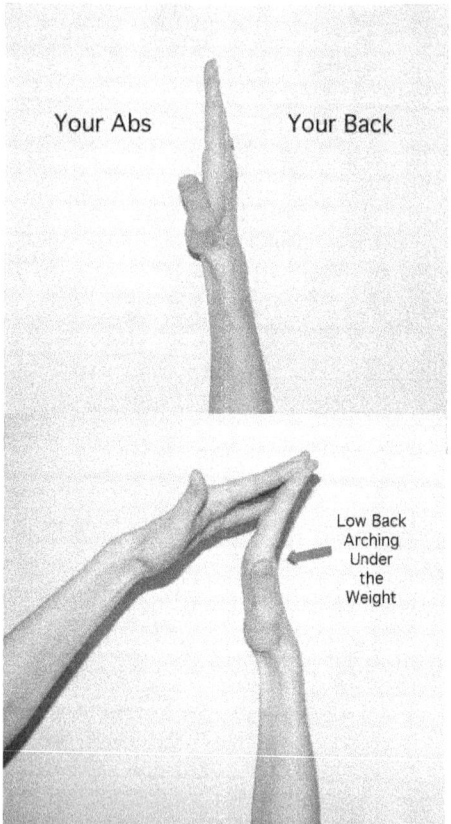

Your Abs   Your Back

2. With your left hand, press the right hand fingers back, bending them as far as they go. Keep the palm upright. Only your fingers arch backward. See and feel the pinched and folded-back crease at the knuckle joints of your right hand.

Low Back Arching Under the Weight

Pushing fingers backward and downward shows how upper body weight pushes backward and downward onto the lower spine when you allow hyperlordosis. The stretched palm of your hand represents your abdomen, with abdominal muscles too long and not pulling to hold you upright and straight.

Bounce against your fingers so that they rock backward repeatedly. Bouncing shows repeated force and compression on your lower back when you walk without using abs to prevent lumbar sway. Now bounce against your fingers quickly and heavily for the concept of the effect of running with lower spine overly angled inward.

3. To represent how your abdominal muscles control spinal angle, and prevent hyperlordosis (swayback), try the following:

With your left hand still pressing the right fingers backward, use muscles in the palm of your right hand to straighten your right hand against the push of your left. Your fingers come back up into a straight line. That is how you need to use abs to control your posture when standing.

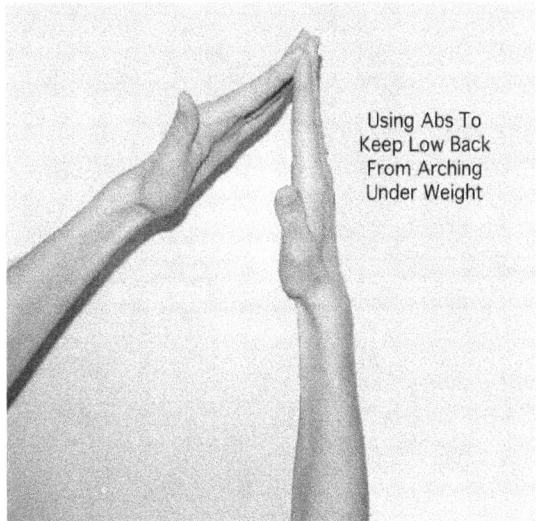

Using Abs To Keep Low Back From Arching Under Weight

Tightening muscles, or strengthening them, does not change positioning. Using the muscles to move the spine is how you prevent the cause of this kind of pain.

Now you know how abdominal muscles are supposed to work to prevent overly large lower spine inward curve (hyperlordosis) that creates back pain. You use abdominal muscles to pull your spine forward enough to straighten from a backward lean to vertical, and return to neutral spine.

Ab Exercises And Core Strengthening Don't Automatically Change Posture, Lumbar Angle, or Lower Back Pain

A common belief is that strengthening muscles changes posture. After spending time and money on strengthening, people often wind up as stronger with the same poor posture. Unhealthy spine position injures no matter how strong you are. Strengthening doesn't make you move.

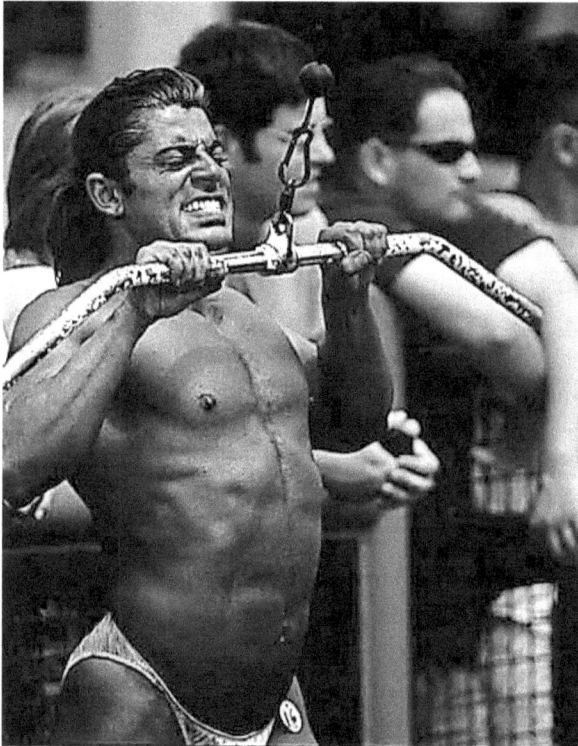

In the photograph above, the abdominal muscles may look strong, however spine angle is still injurious (and silly-looking) hyperlordosis. Strengthening does not create movement to change posture. You create needed movement yourself.

If you strengthen arm muscles, for example, the stronger muscles don't automatically make you hold your arm in the air, or "support" your arm. In the same way, strengthening abdominal muscles does not make them move or support your back. You must deliberately use abdominal muscles (and other muscles, including back muscles) to move your position from injurious to healthy position. For that reason, doing crunches, yoga, and rehab exercises without stopping hyperlordosis does not often work as hoped.

No matter how muscular you are, or how many crunches you have done, you can still slouch into painful swayback. Abdominal muscle use is conscious, deliberate use to move your spine from arched to neutral, like using any other voluntary muscles to move any other part of your body.

Doing abdominal and core exercises is not like getting a shot of penicillin. It does not fix the problem—the bad habits that cause the pain. Using abdominal muscles is like toilet training. You need to learn what to do, make your mistakes until you remember, then hold it even when you don't feel like it.

The rest of Part I shows how to apply The Ab Revolution to fix spine position during everyday life to stop pain. Then use Part II to learn healthy core and whole body strengthening and stretching using neutral spine. Part II also includes how to change the pictured "pull-down" exercise from hyperlordosis to neutral spine, for stronger and more effective core and body exercise.

How to Prevent Back Pain From Hyperlordosis During Walking and Running

Hyperlordosis is a major, but often overlooked, cause of lower back pain during and after walking and running. Pain often goes away with sitting, bending over, or lying down with knees bent. People are often mistakenly told the problem is impact, and told to give up favorite activities. The cause of pain is not impact, which in certain amounts is healthy for bones and body systems, but large inward lumbar curve.

A slight inward curve in the lower back functions as a spring for shock absorption, and keeps forces distributed evenly on discs. Exaggerating the curve allows upper body weight to painfully pinch soft tissue, and joints of the lumbar spine called facets. Allowing the spine to slouch in hyperlordosis also decreases shock absorption and reduces power and speed.

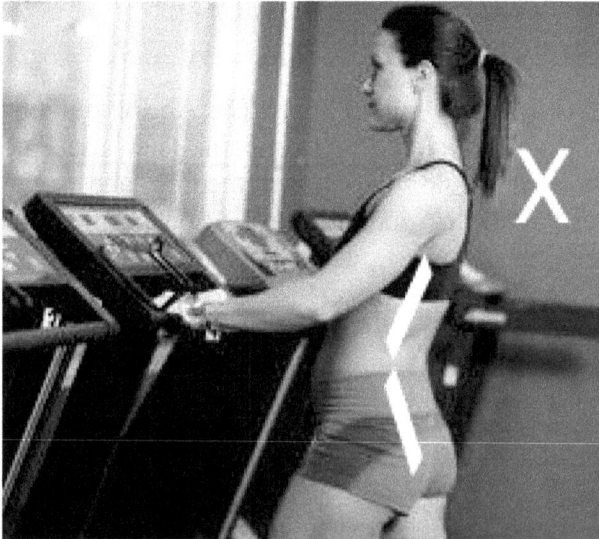

Hyperlordosis. Unhealthful posture. Anterior hip tilt (belt line downward in front) and thoracic lean-back (upper body leans backward).

If you feel you must lean over or sit to relieve lower back discomfort when walking or running, check for hyperlordosis. The cure is not to stop activity, or lean over forward, but to stop the painful posture that causes it. To do that, tuck the pelvis to vertical. Prevent the upper body from leaning backward. Use neutral spine.

If you aren't sure how to move to neutral, use the earlier section, "A Few Ways to Fix Hyperlordosis and Learn Neutral Spine."

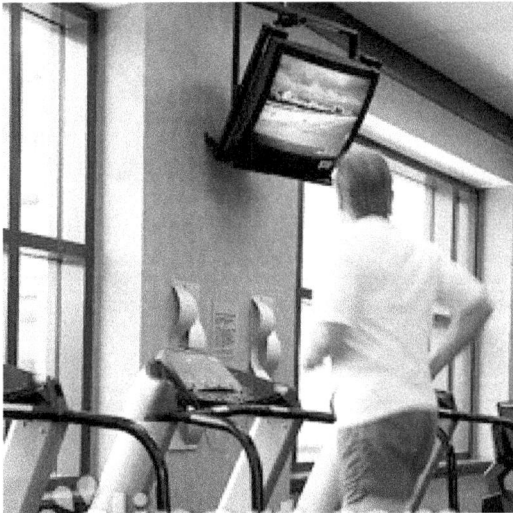

Neutral spine. Torso upright. Hip is level and pelvis vertical.
Don't be fooled by a shirt hem alone. Check actual bodyline.

Treadmill running does not use muscle patterns needed for real terrain. It does not train you how to run in actual situations. Learn how to push a real surface with your own leg muscles rather than having an artificial device burn fuel to push it for you. Learn to run on uneven and changing surfaces. Get out in fresh air and sunshine, or various weather conditions that help condition the body to withstand heat and cold. Get away from a television playing gossip and exploiting tragedies for ratings.

For better health, walk and run outside in healthy sunlight and fresh air rather than a treadmill. These are two major overlooked factors in physical and mental health.

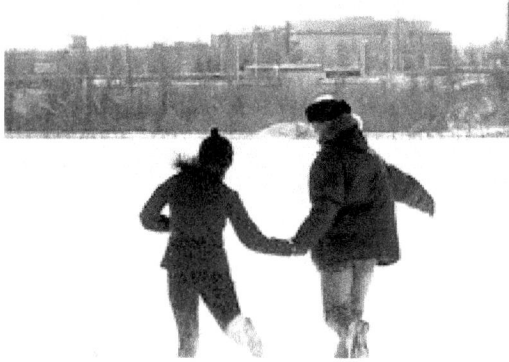

How to Prevent Back Pain From Hyperlordosis During Walking In High Heeled Shoes, and on "Tip-Toe"

A common statement is that high heels make you arch your back. They do not make you, however it is common to increase lumbar curve to help balance when wearing heeled shoes or when standing "tip-toe." The painful, unhealthful increased inward spine curve is preventable.

The photos below show barefoot practice. One foot is forward for two reasons, so that you can see both feet, and because that is part of how you walk, while wearing heels or not. You can practice in bare feet or wearing shoes. Then apply what you learned when wearing heeled shoes.

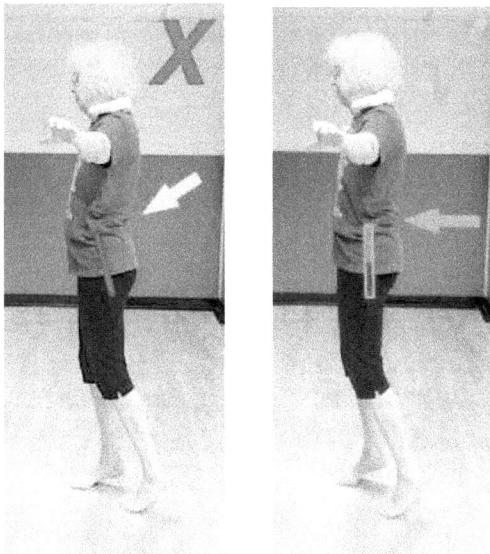

Left: Hyperlordosis. Anterior pelvic tilt, Upper body is leaning back. Right: Pelvis corrected to vertical. The upper body is still leaning back slightly. When you do this, keep upper body vertical.

1. Rise to stand on the ball of the foot (commonly called "tip-toe" "half-toe" and "standing on your toes" even though you are not all the way onto the toes.)

2. Notice if you increase lumbar arch. Notice if you learn the upper body backwards or tilt the pelvis.

3. Correct to neutral spine. Bring upper body forward until vertical. Tuck pelvis under until vertical.

If you are not sure how to control spine position wearing heeled shoes, go to Part I, "A Few Ways to Fix Hyperlordosis and Learn Neutral Spine." Try the standing methods while standing on the ball of the foot with heels off the floor, simulating wearing high-heeled shoes. Then try walking on the ball of the foot (heels raised) in neutral spine.

High heels may not allow healthy foot mechanics or toe spacing. They may not have good padding and may painfully press the feet. They may be a trip hazard, make balance harder, and impede speed and mobility. However, they do not "make" you increase lumbar arch. Wearing them is more work to stand healthfully neutral, but that is what abdominal muscles are for.

How to Prevent Lower Back Pain When Reaching Overhead

Notice if you lean your upper body backward or tip your hip forward when reaching up. These actions increase lower spine arch.

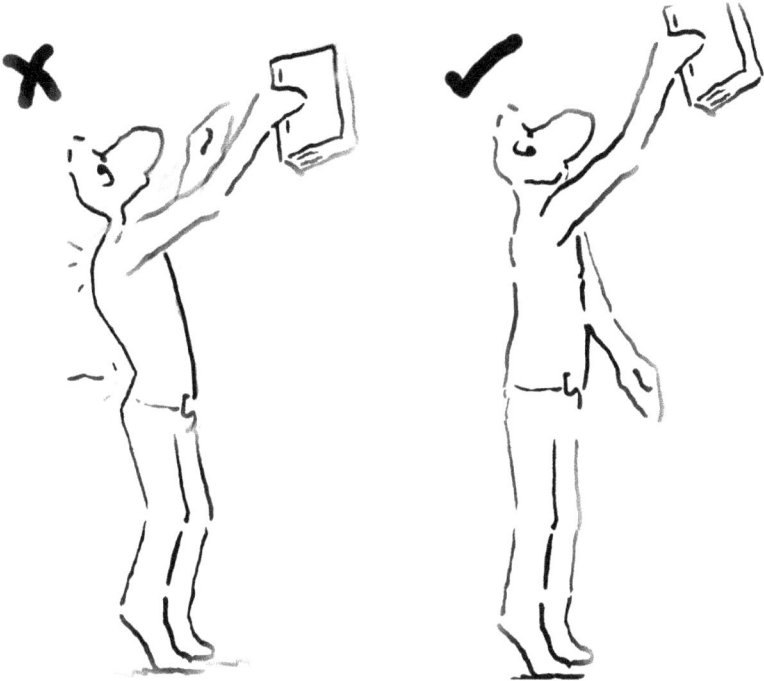

Left: Hyperlordosis. Pelvis tilted forward. Upper body tilted backward.
Right: Neutral spine. Upper back and pelvis vertical.

1. If the pelvis tilts forward, swing it under until vertical. If you learn the upper body backward, bring your upper body forward until upright. Use abdominal muscles as if you were beginning a crunch of both the upper and lower body, but not curling shoulders or neck forward.

2. You may notice that your arm doesn't reach as high, at first. While holding tucked, straight spine and hip position, get more range from the shoulder, not spine, for better shoulder stretch.

Notice other people who allow their lower spine to increase in lumbar curve when reaching for shelves, packages, groceries, lifting a baby or child, talking a photograph, combing hair, pulling off shirts, at the gym to lift weights, and everywhere. Use that to remind yourself to identify and stop doing that yourself.

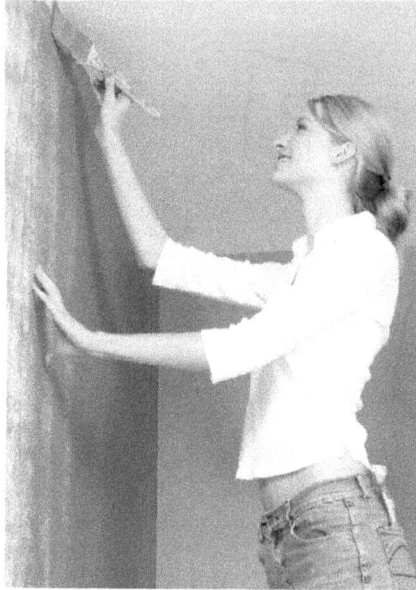

Hyperlordosis during reaching, pictured above, is a common cause of lower back pain after activities.

Don't confuse leaning back in hyperlordosis with good shoulder range overhead. A common scenario is someone with shoulder pain who is asked by the health provider to reach overhead. The person leans backward to point the arm straight overhead. If this is missed, the person may be told shoulder range is normal when the shoulder did not extend as much as it seemed.

Keep neutral spine when reaching and lifting overhead. You will get more range of motion from the shoulder, more exercise for abdominal muscles, and a direct way to stop the kind of lower back pain that comes from leaning backward and tilting the pelvis during reaching activities.

How to use neutral spine when lifting overhead

1. Check if you learn your upper body backward or tilt your hip as you raise arms.

2. To reduce too much lumbar curve, flex the lower spine as if beginning a crunch until upper body comes forward until vertical and belt line becomes level.

3. Feel effort shift to your abdominal muscles. Done correctly, pressure in the lower back from hyperlordosis should be gone with no new pain substituted.

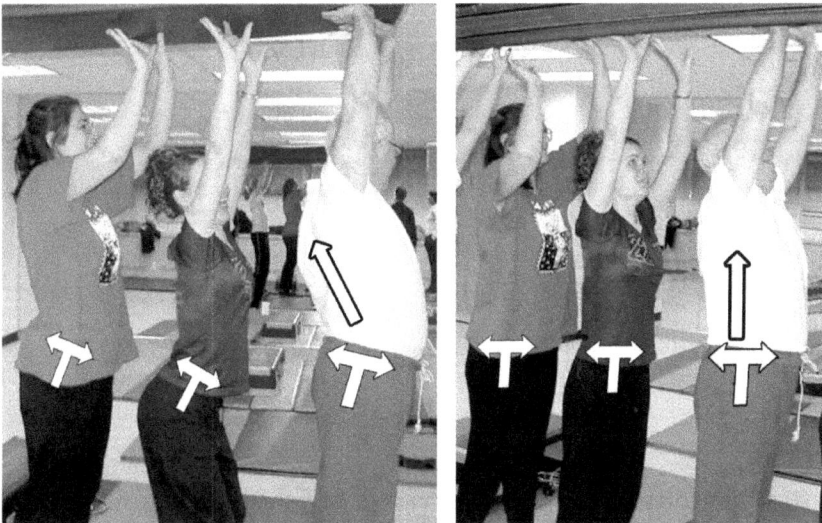

Left: Hyperlordosis. Pelvis tilts forward in each subject. Upper body leans backward. Right: Neutral spine. Beltline level. Upper body is vertical.

If you aren't sure how to move to neutral, use the earlier section, "A Few Ways to Fix Hyperlordosis and Learn Neutral Spine." More about reaching up with neutral spine for exercise and lifting weights is in Part II.

How to Prevent Lower Back Pain When Carrying Loads in Front — Anterior Loads

When carrying things in front of the body, it is common to lean the upper body backward (thoracic lean-back) to offset the weight. The pelvis may also tilt forward (anterior tilt). Resulting increased lumbar curve shifts weight of the load to the lower spine, and off the abdominal muscles. Hyperlordosis makes carrying loads feel easier because it is less work for the muscles. The result is fewer calories burned, less exercise, and more painful angle of the spine.

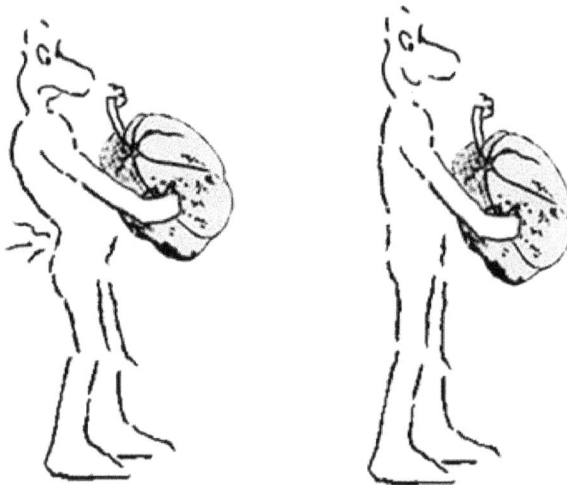

Left: Hyperlordosis. Anterior pelvic tilt and thoracic lean-back. Right: Neutral spine. More abdominal work. No injurious spine angle.

1. Instead of leaning backward, keep the upper body vertical. Don't overdo by rounding or leaning forward.

2. Change a tilted pelvis to vertical. Don't overly tuck the hip, push it forward, or tighten any muscles.

3. Feel how the large lumbar curve lessens to a smaller neutral curve. Pressure in the lower back from hyperlordosis should immediately stop. No new pain should be substituted.

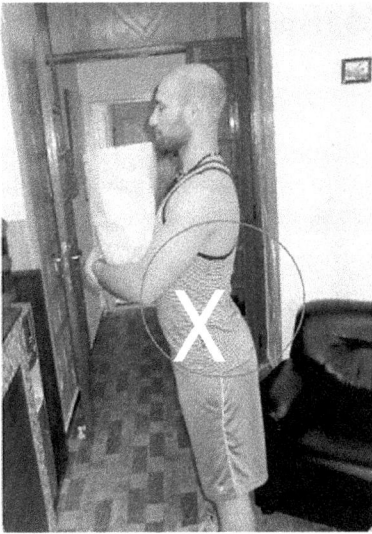

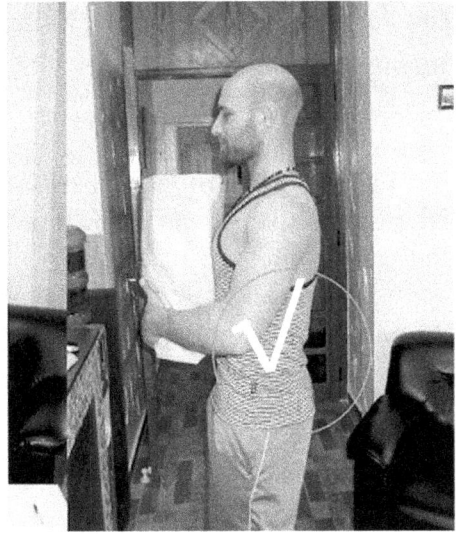

Left: Thoracic lean-back is easily missed when it is from an already forward position, giving the illusion of aligned upper body when it is not. Right: Neutral spine.

When carrying or lifting any load in front, from groceries, to a chair, to dumbbells and hand weights, to a pregnancy or a baby in arms or a front carrier, don't lean to offset the load. Maintain upright upper body and neutral spine against the pull of the load. You will feel abdominal muscles working to do this. It gives free core exercise, and reduces wear on the lower back soft tissues and joints called facets. If you aren't sure how to move to neutral, use the earlier section, "A Few Ways to Fix Hyperlordosis and Learn Neutral Spine."

It is not necessary to lean back to offset a load. It may be tempting to lean, letting the lower spine take the weight. Instead, get free arm and abdominal exercise. Save leaning for emergencies, for loads far heavier than your strength allows. See Part II to learn healthy strengthening so you can be safer in emergencies, and have fun doing more.

How to Prevent Lower Back Pain from Hyperlordosis During Pregnancy

One major source of back pain during pregnancy is hyperlordosis. Hyperlordosis is not caused by a pregnant belly, or a beer belly, or any load carried in front of the body. It is from leaning the upper body backward or tilting the pelvis to offset the weight, instead of holding neutral spine position against the load.

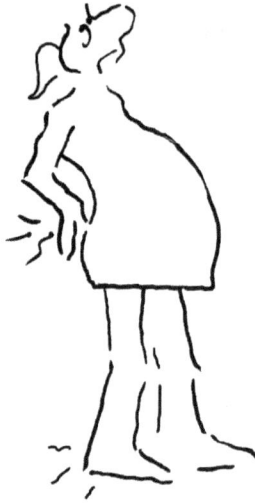

Too much inward lumbar curve, pictured above, can be corrected to neutral spine during pregnancy, the same as during any other time.

It is not true that the only way to balance a load in front of you is to lean backward or tilt the pelvis. It is the job of your abdominal muscles to offset the weight. They will only do that if you deliberately use them to hold neutral spine against the weight and make it a habit.

Hyperlordosis is not an unavoidable consequence of pregnancy. Of all times to use abdominal muscles to prevent change in back posture and the back pain that results, this is the time.

If you aren't sure how to move your spine to neutral, use the earlier section, "A Few Ways to Fix Hyperlordosis and Learn Neutral Spine."

How To Prevent Lower Back Pain When Carrying Loads On Your Back

It is not true that carrying shoulder bags or a backpack "makes you arch your back" or lean to the back or side. You may be allowing your spine to slouch under the weight of a bag, or you may lean to offset the weight. Instead, keep both upper body and pelvis vertical against the pull of the weight of the pack. The pack becomes a built-in core workout plus pain relief.

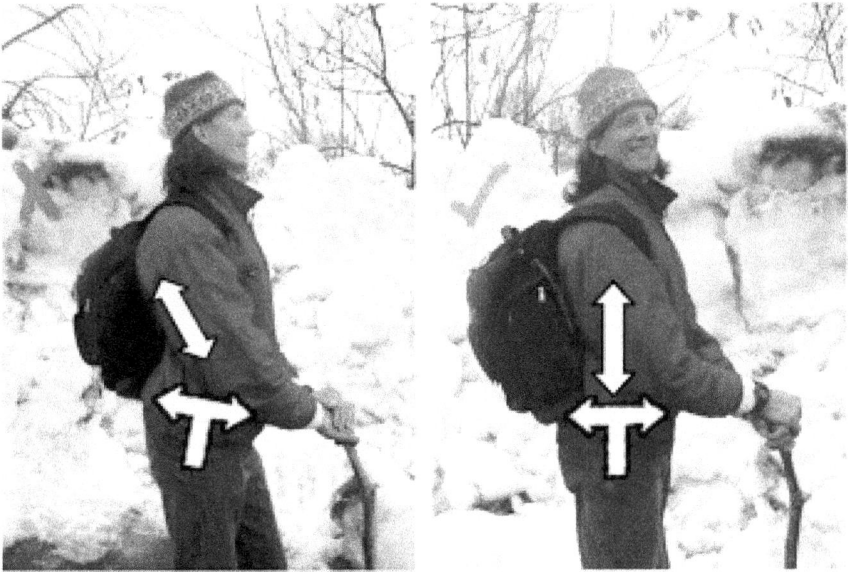

Left: Hyperlordosis. Anterior pelvic tilt and thoracic lean-back. Weight of the backpack shifted to lower spine. Right: Level beltline. Vertical upper body. Abdominal muscles hold neutral spine against the load.

To practice how to change hyperlordosis to healthy spine position under a posterior load:

1. Stand wearing any heavy bag or backpack. Look in a mirror to see yourself from the side-view. See and feel if you lean your upper body backward, or tilt your pelvis, or push it forward.

2. If you lean the upper body backward (thoracic lean-back), pull forward to upright position. Don't round the shoulders. Feel your torso straighten against the pull of the bag.

3. If your pelvis tilts so that your beltline comes downward in front, tuck under until vertical. Do not push your pelvis forward. Keep in place while you change the anterior tilt to a vertical position.

4. If you push the entire pelvis forward, pictured below, bring the pelvis back and upper body forward until both are vertical.

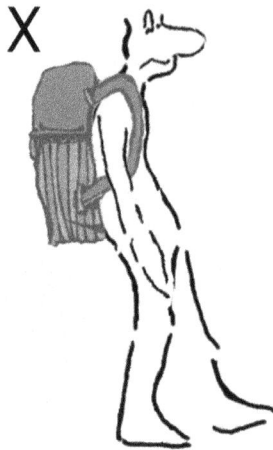

Done correctly, you should feel back pain from hyperlordosis disappear, and effort shift to your abdominal muscles as soon as you change from swayback to neutral.

People go to a gym to use an "ab machine" to pull forward to work their muscles. Any posterior load you carry, from backpacks to baby carriers can become a free, built-in workout and pain-prevention trainer if you use neutral spine against the pull of the load.

If you aren't sure how to move to neutral spine, use the earlier section, "A Few Ways to Fix Hyperlordosis and Learn Neutral Spine."

Shoulder Bags And Babies Carried On The Hip

Hyperlordosis pain is common from letting the spine slouch to the side under the weight of carried items, instead of holding upright position using core muscles.

Even if you don't have scoliosis, which is an abnormal and often painful sideways spine curve, you can create and enforce a similar curve from habitual bad positioning and movement mechanics. This is preventable.

When holding packages on your hip, a baby, or carrying a heavy handbag on one shoulder or hip, notice if you are leaning. Straighten against the sideways pull of whatever you carry. The straightening action uses your oblique (side) abdominal muscles).

How to Prevent Back Pain From Hyperlordosis During Swimming and Scuba Diving

Although swimming is a common prescription for back pain, it is also common to increase back pain through unhealthful spine and shoulder positioning. It is not true that swimming the front crawl, or other strokes on the front, "makes you arch your back." However, it is common to allow it, which is why sending back pain patients to go swimming may not stop their back pain. Check if you are swimming in hyperlordosis (swayback) and correct it.

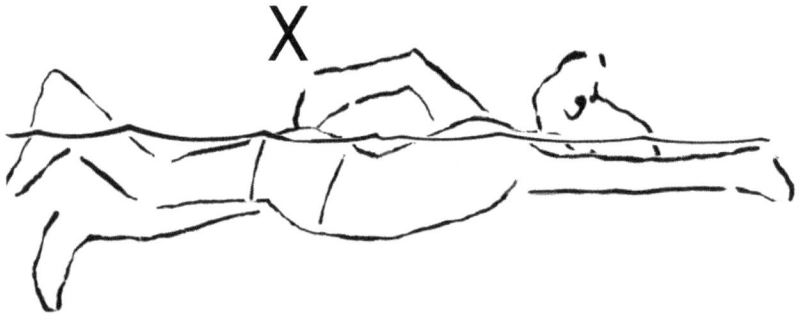

Swayback (hyperlordosis), pictured above, is a common contributor to lower back pain from swimming and scuba diving.

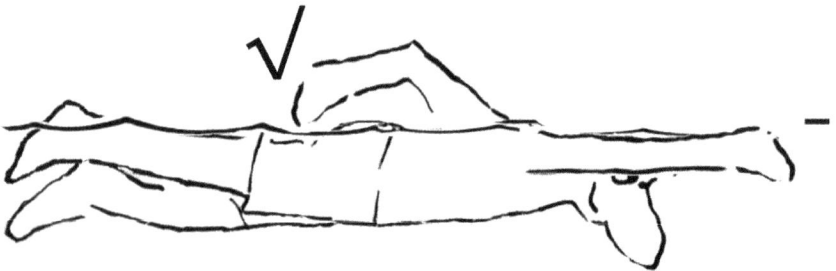

Neutral spine for swimming and scuba diving improves streamline, and prevents pain from hyperlordosis. Head position varies according to stroke or what you are looking at.

Wearing scuba tanks doesn't make you arch your back or use swayback posture. Not using your abdominal muscles to counter the pull, allowing your lower spine to increase inward curve, is the problem.

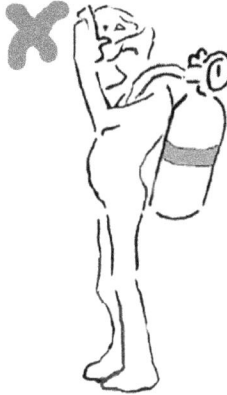

1. Check if you allow swayback while wearing tanks, either standing or during your dive. Straighten to neutral spine. Straighten the pelvis using a pelvic tilt or tucking motion if needed, and bring the upper body vertical and upright.

2. Breathe. Feel your abdominal muscles hold position against the weight of the tanks but do not tighten your abdominal or other muscles. Feel a better streamline in the water.

3. When standing with tanks, don't lean backwards or push your hips forward. Stand upright.

Done correctly, you will feel your abdominal muscles working against the pull of the load. Lower back pain from hyperlordosis should be gone, and no new pain should be substituted.

If you aren't sure how to stop hyperlordosis, use the earlier section, "A Few Ways to Fix Hyperlordosis and Learn Neutral Spine."

How To Stop Back Pain From Hyperlordosis From Golf

Lower back pain with golf is usually attributed to twisting, since that is when many people feel pain. However, besides repeated forward bending, common for retrieving golf shots and equipment, a main overlooked source of lower back pain from golf is hyperlordosis during the swing (and standing and carrying gear). Increasing inward curve in the lower back during the swing pinches spine joints called facets, and surrounding soft tissue. Injury process increases from rapid-onset, forceful hyperlordosis on each swing.

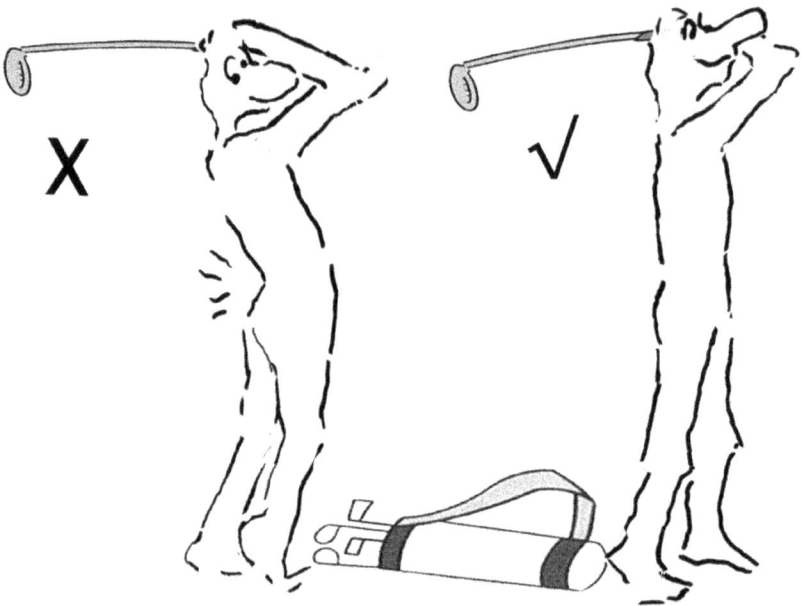

It is not the case that the only way to get full swing range or power is by hyperlordosis. With neutral spine, the effort of the swing shifts to abdominal muscles. Used right, it gives a powerful swing with greater range that comes from the hip, entire spine, and shoulders, not one overly compressed lumbar segment.

When Your Lower Back Hurts to Lie Flat Without A Pillow

Three main areas, when tight, make it uncomfortable to lie flat: anterior hip, lumbar, and chest.

Anterior Hip. Hip flexors are muscles that bend your leg forward (flex) at the hip. Tight hip flexors can't lengthen enough to extend legs straight. Without sufficient resting length at the anterior hip to allow the legs to lie flat, the spine pulls into a pinched angle. When lying on the back, a pillow under the knees (and bent knees for exercise) reduces lumbar curve while knees are bent, and is mistaken for a fix, but perpetuates shortened muscles. The answer is not to take away the pillow but the need for it, which is tightness. Note the bent hip in the illustrations below. Needed range comes from the lower spine, pulled into arch, pinching the lower back, making it ache.

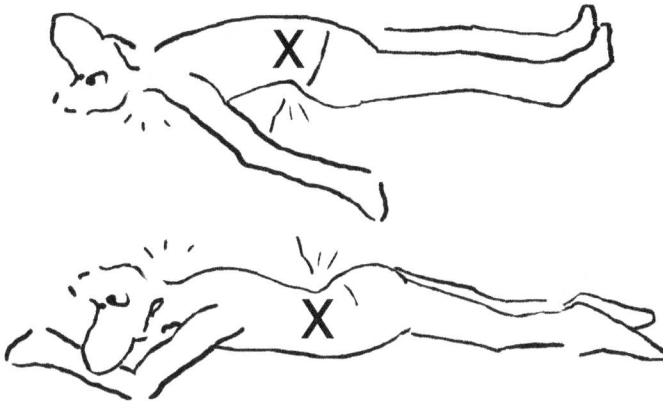

The same pain from too large lumbar curve can occur lying face down. Mistaken beliefs arose that lying face down is bad for the back, or pain is from a condition or weakness, or that you need special beds, when pain is from preventable tightness (unless you sleep face down in a hammock). Many people are told never to sleep face down, even if it is what they love. Some would prefer it, if it didn't hurt. Some are told to bring knees to chest in the morning as "antidote" for resulting pain, when stopping the cause by stretching tight areas to stop hyperlordosis is healthier, and prevents the pain in the first place.

When the front of the hip has healthy resting length, in most cases, you would be able to comfortably lie face up and face down. Then you will no longer have the pain or need the pillow.

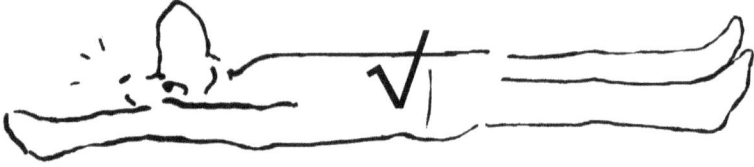

A Few Stretches for Tight Anterior Hip
For the following, if you aren't sure how to move to neutral, use the earlier section, "A Few Ways to Fix Hyperlordosis and Learn Neutral Spine."

Standing lunge is a combination hip stretch and leg strengthener. It retrains one way to bend for things in daily life. Stand with feet in whatever width you need for real life bending and enough to get a stretch too. Keep the back foot facing forward not turned. Heel is lifted. Bend both knees, keeping body weight centered. Tip your hip under to reduce lumbar arch. Done right, you'll feel new stretch in the front of the rear leg. The lunge for exercise is described more in Part II.

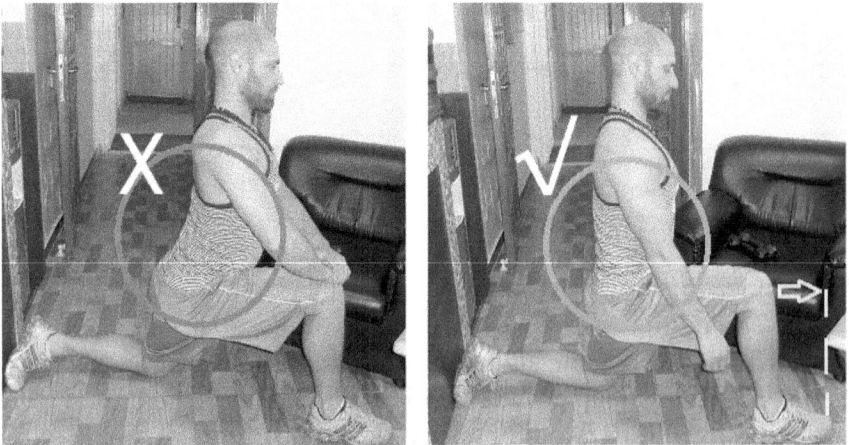

Left: Hyperlordosis. Large lumbar sway. Hip tilted. Hands on front knee. Right: Neutral lunge. Hip tucked. Not leaning on hand. Increased anterior hip and lumbar stretch.

Stretching front hip muscles over a ball, bed, or any object. To stretch backward (extend) over an exercise ball, pillow, or other object, and for hanging legs over the end of a bed, check if the motion you get is from arching your back instead of from the front of the hip, as intended. Increasing lumbar arch is counterproductive to what you are trying to do. The purpose of the stretch is to lengthen and "unbend" (extend) the hip and upper back.

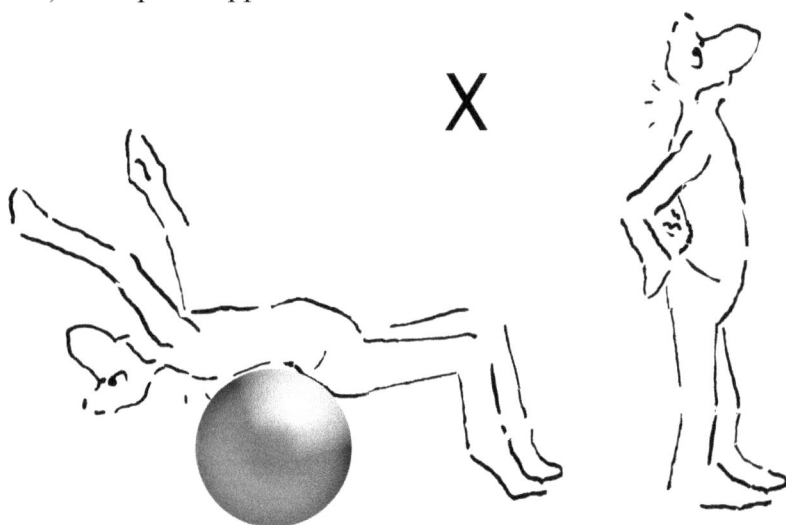

Don't stretch with the same hyperlordosis you are trying to fix.

Place the ball (or other object) under your hip, not lower back, to stretch the front of the hip. If you feel pinching in your lower back, tuck your hip to reduce the arch. Done right, you will feel the stretch move to your front hip, and pinching disappear from your spine. Done right, it will feel good and be healthy and useful.

Standing quadriceps (thigh) stretch. Reduce lower back arch by tucking the pelvis to neutral. Done right, you will feel the stretch move to your quadriceps and front muscles of your hip. Don't bring the knee forward. The point is to lengthen anterior muscles, not shorten them by bending your leg forward at the hip. This stretch is described in full in Part II, "How to Use Abs For Neutral Spine For Quadriceps Stretching."

Notice Tightness Habits. Watch for flexed (bent forward) hip by watching clothing side seams and belt line. Keep side seam vertical, not tilted from waist to hip. Belt line from a side view should be horizontal. If the belt tips down in front because you stand arched, (not because you wear your belt that way) tuck your hip under until neutral. Don't push the pelvis forward. Neutral spine, taught throughout this book is a built-in natural anterior stretch.

Why Do Anterior Muscles Shorten?

Many people keep their hip bent forward at the crease where the leg meets the body during most of their life. They stand and walk with the pelvis tilted, sleep with a pillow under their knees, do mainly flexion exercises, bend forward for most of their yoga, bend their knees and hip (shortened hip muscle) to do exercises in the belief bending knees protects the back, then sit the rest of the time. See more about benefit of keeping legs straight for core exercise in Part II, *Isometric Abs* drill. Sitting is blamed for tightness, but lack of length also comes from not using healthy length to stand and move in neutral spine the rest of the day. Much conventional "fitness" and pop exercise encourages this unhealthy, unattractive bad posture. Exercises and activities of daily living (ADLs) with the hip bent (flexed) shortens it, and tightness makes flexed posture feel normal.

Tight Chest and Upper Body

Tight front chest muscles make round-shouldered position feel normal. Round-shouldered positioning keeps the front muscles shortened, in a cycle of shortening and tightening. Upper back muscles overly lengthen. Many traditional stretches use rounding forward. Avoid them, along with pulling one arm over your chest in front, which further encourages round-shouldered position. It is so counterproductive, it can be called, "The Stretch You Need The Least."

If upper body and shoulders are so tight that you cannot stand straight without arching your back or craning your neck, try stretching the front muscles of your chest (pectoral muscles). One quick, chest (pectoral) stretch is to closely face a wall and brace the inside of one bent elbow against the wall out to one side. Turn your feet and body away from the elbow using the wall to brace and pull the arm behind your body. Done right, you will feel the stretch in the front chest muscles of the stretched arm only, with no pinching in the shoulder joint. Use stretches that extend your upper spine backward in healthy ways, not forward. A good stretch book resource is listed at the end of Part III.

Lumbar (Lower Back) Shortening and Tightness
Hyperlordosis holds lumbar structures at shortened length. Eventually, structures become too shortened and tight to comfortably stand without hyperlordosis, or lie down without pillows holding you in bent positions. Lumbar stretching would be needed.

Bending forward to touch toes from a stand or sit often feels good to those who tighten the lower back with habitual swayback, but are not healthy over the long term for discs. See the following section on Flexion and Discs. Other lumbar stretches are healthier:

- Use good bending for everything you crouch and bend for. Use a neutral spine squat, not hyperlordotic squat. See Part II for good bending using squats.

- Low squats are sometimes called "Asian sitting." The slight rounding along the entire spine during full low squat is not injurious for most, and gives needed, built-in, daily stretch. Ability to rest comfortably in low squat increases as your flexibility increases by using habitual good bending with partial squats. To help learn low squats, hold a support in front of you. Keep both heels down and lean back as you squat as low as you can. If you keep heels down, you will feel a good stretch on both the lower spine and Achilles tendon.

- Use neutral spine for daily life. It gives built in lumbar stretch.

- More stretches are in the stretching book listed at the end of Part III.

A Little About Disc Injury and Flexion

Chronic excess inward lumbar curve (hyperlordosis) is a cause of much facet joint and soft tissue back pain. The opposite, too much bending forward, (flexion) is more associated with disc injury, and also muscle pain. Most conventional core exercises and common stretches are flexion, (bending forward). They are counterproductive for most people after a day of sitting. Flexion doesn't cancel the damage of hyperlordosis. even if it feels good for the moment. Each can accumulate damage.

With the small normal inward lumbar curve, vertebrae line up on each other like stacks of cups, with distributed pressure on discs from front to back. Rounding forward (and some side bends) unequally sheer and load discs. Chronic repeated weighted forward bending eventually damages discs. This is the herniation process.

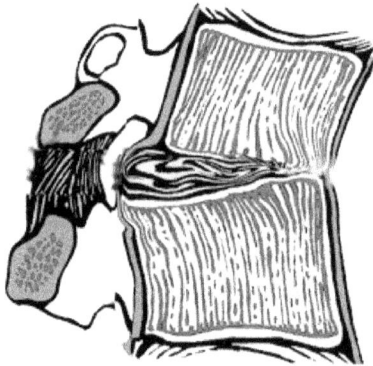

Side view facing right, of two spine bones (vertebrae) and one disc between them. Habitual bending forward for toe touching, weight lifting, and picking things up, and sideways (for example, yoga triangles) can slowly, mechanically, bulge the discs rearward.

After years of weighted forward bending, a disc can finally degenerate and bulge enough to hurt. It feels sudden, but like a heart attack from unhealthy lifestyle, it was building over many years. Disc herniation is an injury, not a disease, and is easily preventable.

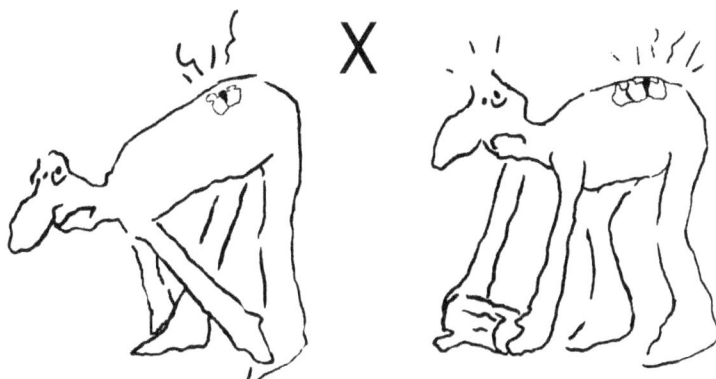

Years of forward (and side) bending can sheer and deform discs
enough to degenerate and herniate them.

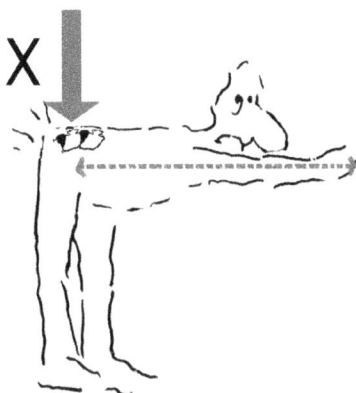

Straight back is higher force on discs; because of
longer distance to fulcrum of spine.

Bending forward with straight back, sometimes called hip hinge, makes another problem of a longer lever and higher disc force than with an upright bend or bending with rounded back. It is a small back exercise but not worth the extra wear on discs. Resting arms and upper body on something is one change, if you use it as a brief stretch. However there are better back and hamstrings stretches, see More Resources, at the end of this book.

Side bends for yoga have been found in some studies to have more herniating force on discs than front bends. Holding triangles for more than two to three seconds increases sheer. By contrast, a few brief side-to-side motions, like a slow windshield wiper, can give discs needed range of motion and a brief squeezing that helps move nutrition and wastes. Holding long side bends is not healthy for the discs. Side bends are also known to increase impingement on the hip socket. Many practitioners bend sideways in ways that jam the ball of the upper leg bone into the hip socket. If you do triangles, use them as a one or two second stretch, or a one second transition move to something else that is healthier.

It is not true that "discs only get worse." They get worse only if you keep pushing them out. With healthy mechanics, you can stay active without pain while they heal. They can get better.

Almost any movement for exercise can feel good in the short term, even if damage is accruing. Neutral spine exercise avoids both problems. For healthy bending and lifting, use a partial squat. Healthy squat is done with neutral spine and upright torso. Healthy bending shifts load off your discs and soft tissue and onto the leg, hip, and back muscles. Keep your knees back over the feet, rather than sliding forward. For neck health, instead of only lifting the chin and bending back at one neck segment, get more range from the upper back, keeping neck in relaxed neutral position.

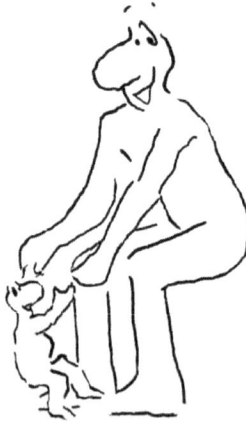

Neutral spine bending is healthy bending for spine discs and all the rest of you. Use neutral spine squatting instead of increasing lumbar arch. If you aren't sure how to move to neutral spine, use the section, "A Few Ways to Fix Hyperlordosis and Learn Neutral Spine."

Disc Injury and Hyperlordosis

Hyperlordosis was not previously thought of as a herniating force on discs. The major factor in producing disc injury is too much forward bending, briefly covered in the previous section.

For someone with a disc already herniated, hyperlordosis can often pinch already protruded discs, adding pain to the separate problem of the disc injury, and may add to the herniation process. For these people, learning to stop standing in hyperlordosis often quickly reduces their disc pain. Stopping main causes of disc injury still needs addressing (bad bending, bad sitting, bad exercises). Occasionally, discs may protrude in directions that make neutral spine uncomfortable. Don't force neutral, and concentrate first on letting discs reduce. The previous section describes briefly, with more in the resources listed at the end of Part III.

New work is finding that hyperlordosis may be a potential mechanism to directly shift and degenerate, or contribute to shifting or sheering discs. The diagram below shows disc injury from the exaggerated lumbar hyperlordosis, common in pop fitness.

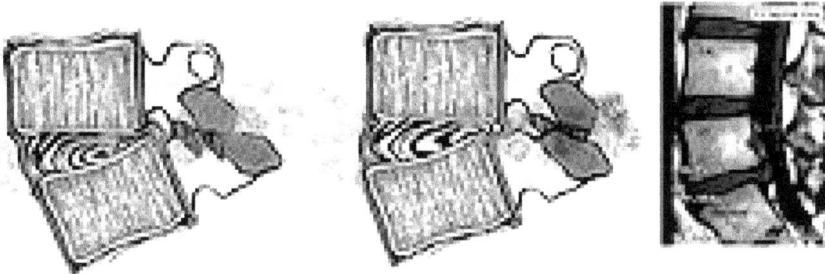

Above Left and Center: Drawings of two ways you can stand in hyperlordosis (antero and retro), and the results on the discs over time. Right: MRI scan generally comparable to center drawing, shows an already bulging disc pinched by vertebrae from the hyperlordotic posture.

Can Someone With Herniated Discs In The Neck Or Back, Osteoporosis, Upper Crossed Syndrome, Hernia Use The Ab Revolution?

Disc Injury and Osteoporosis

The Ab Revolution is not a specific method to fix disc injury. The Ab Revolution is designed to stop pain from hyperlordosis (which may occur along with disc injury or separately). One of several benefits to discs is that The Ab Revolution does not use forward rounding or bending for exercise, which has been found to be a large factor in disc damage. Forward bending of conventional abdominal and core training (crunches, curl-ups, V-sits, "hundreds," and others that bend the spine and hip forward) over time puts degenerative and herniating forces on discs, reinforces rounding spine posture, and are not a good idea for anyone with rounding or fractures from osteoporosis. The Ab Revolution teaches how to straighten the spine to healthful position at the same time as including strengthening for major sites of osteoporosis, the upper back, wrist, and femoral neck (leg bone where it meets the hip).

Upper Back Pain

A habitually rounded upper body posture is a large factor in upper back pain that sometimes was given the name "Upper Crossed Syndrome." People who stand in hyperlordosis by leaning their upper body backward often overly-round the upper back without knowing it. Often they think they are bringing their shoulders back "for good posture" when they are actually bringing the entire upper body backwards. Telling this population to "bring their shoulders back" compounds their problem. Instead, they need to bring the upper body forward as a unit to vertical, and straighten ("unround") their upper spine. It is usually the upper spine, not shoulders, which round too much and need correcting. Isolating the upper back with exercises to treat pain doesn't stop the source of the pain. Ab Revolution actively retrains you to identify and correct the involved segments, and stop the cause of pain.

Abdominal Hernia and Diastasis Recti

Hopeful reports have been coming in from patients with abdominal hernia and diastasis recti (abdominal muscle separation), who say that while flexion-based abdominal exercises hurt or worsen abdominal hernia pain and bulging, they can use Ab Revolution, even the more strenuous, without pain or increased bulging. Use your own judgment and don't use anything that hurts or worsens the situation. Check back as data accrue.

For all your concerns, check with your health providers. Work sensibly to increase your health and physical abilities, and be able to do more, not less.

Stop Back Pain When Sitting - Not Rounded, Not Arched

When you sit, check to see if you are rounding forward, or do the opposite, increase inward lumbar curve. Both can hurt after time.

Sitting Too Rounded. Sitting with your back rounded, along with chronic bending forward, can eventually sheer, degenerate, and bulge vertebral discs (disc herniation).

Disc damage is not a disease, even though it is often mistakenly called "disc disease." It is a mechanical injury process, straightforward to prevent and reverse. Discs are living parts that can heal, , usually quickly, if you let them.

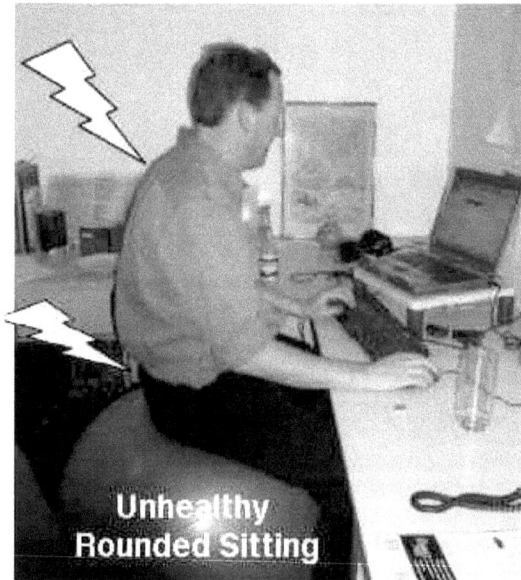

Sitting on a ball does not prevent slouching. Sitting on an exercise ball of any kind will not increase core use, fix pain, or cause you to sit in healthy position.

Swayback Sitting Hurts. Holding a large inward curve does not cancel damage from rounding forward, and can cause its own pain.

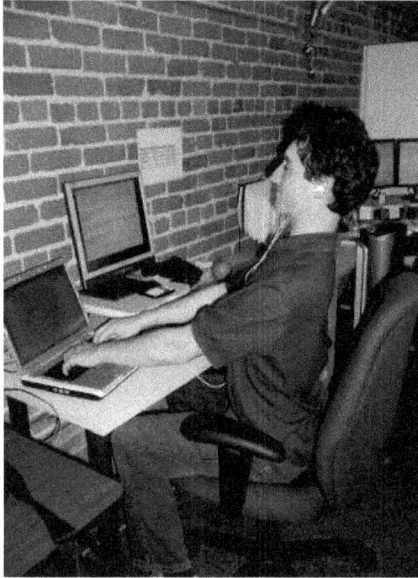

Hyperlordosis during sitting is a common source of tight, tired muscles, and pinched lower spine.

Posture rules for sitting often make more pain. Any rigid tense sitting would hurt. To sit in relaxed, comfortable, healthy way:

1. Check if the back of your chair is concave (rounded outward). Put a *small* soft spacer, often called a "lumbar roll," in concavity of the seat back. A small soft towel (folded not rolled), shirt, or pair of gloves can work as well or better than expensive commercial lumbar rolls.

2. Sit with your hips all the way at the back of the seat. Lean your upper back comfortably against the seat back. Do not round or push your lower back against the roll. If the roll is uncomfortable, it may be too big, or not properly placed, or is made of a hard rigid material. To see approximate size and placement of a lumbar roll, put your own hand or forearm comfortably in the space between your lower back and the seat and lean back comfortably.

3. You should feel relief from pressure on your lower back right away when fixing to relaxed healthy position. If it hurts, it's wrong. Stop and readjust whatever is wrong.

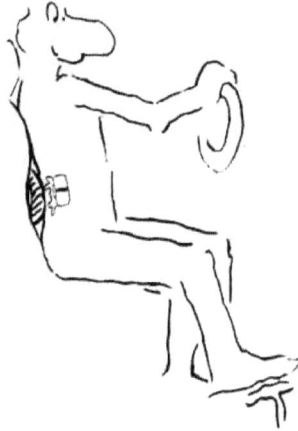

Neutral spine using a lumbar roll. Lean the upper body back against the seat, not the lower back against the roll.

Get up from sitting

Common instructions that sitting is unhealthy because it is sedentary and in bent forward position, often include stretches. Often these stretches are done sitting, even lying down (even more sedentary), and involve the same bent forward hip, back, shoulder, or neck positions as sitting. For example, touching toes, bringing knee to chest, chin to chest, or arm forward over the body.

All Ab Revolution exercises in Part II train how to straighten the body in relaxed healthy ways while getting needed movement. Healthy extension also helps after sitting. Extension stretches and exercises are in Part II.

Reference Sheet For Healthy Bending, Reaching, and Lifting

BAD Bending Hurts Back, Knees, Neck.

GOOD Bending & Lifting Healthy for All

Bad Bending -
Minor back exercise
Increased spine risk

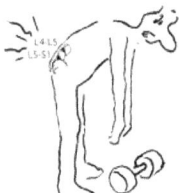

Bad Bending -
Straight spine
INCREASES bad spine force

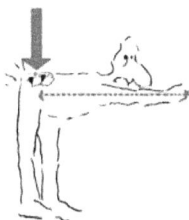

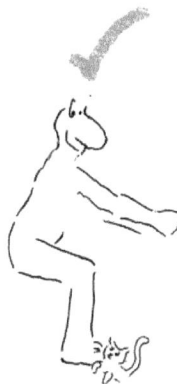

Bad back AND knees AND neck
Knees forward,
Neck bent back
Back rounded forward

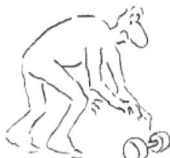

or overarch inward

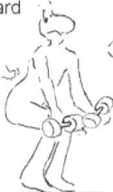

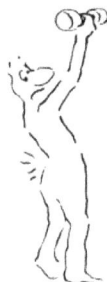

Bad Lifting -
Leaning upper body backward
Hip tilted forward
Too much inward lumbar curve
(hyperlordosis / swayback)
Compresses Lower Spine

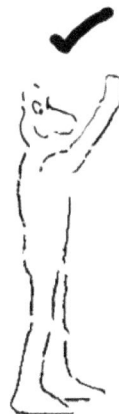

Neutral neck
Neutral spine
Knees over feet

Part II

Ab Revolution™ Exercises for Healthy, Effective, Core and Whole Body Strengthening and Stretching

Key Points Part II

Part II teaches Ab Revolution exercises using neutral spine from simple to challenging for healthy exercise, stretch, and strength. Use Part I to learn neutral spine.

Strength and movement are important to healthy life. However, not all exercise is good for you. Healthy core training uses neutral spine and directly avoids both unhealthful flexion and hyperlordosis.

Ab Revolution teaches core exercise the way needed for real life, and also benefits the rest of your body, for both looks and health.

Getting the overall concepts and applying them broadly with quick improvements is more important and useful than spending time on tiny details.

At first, it may be a surprise to not be able to do many of the Ab Revolution exercises for more than a few seconds. You need specific abdominal strength and endurance to hold healthful position. No wonder posture often sags by the end of the day and muscles ache. Work to increase the time you hold your new healthy spine position with these exercises.

What Is Different About Ab Revolution Exercises?

- Teaches effective abdominal and whole body exercise at the same time as directly retraining spine positioning.

- Trains your muscles and spine in the way you need to stand and move in real life, not only when lying on the floor or "doing exercises."

- Directly retrains hyperlordosis to neutral spine to stop hyperlordosis as a major cause of back pain. Teaches abdominal and core exercises in neutral spine for better exercise without forward bending, to stop other kinds of pain. Chronic forward bending is a contributor to bad posture as a habit, muscular back pain, disc damage, and sciatica.

- Dispels myths about abdominal and core training. For example, why you don't tighten, or "suck them in" or "press navel to spine." Tightening does not change injurious spine position or put you into healthy position. You cannot breath in well or move properly when you hold your abdomen tightly. Another myth is that you must keep your knees bent during exercises to "keep your back in proper position." If it were true that you have to bend your knees to protect your back, how are you supposed to stand up and walk away? It is not knees that position your lower spine, but abdominal muscles. The Ab Revolution teaches you specifically how to use your abdominal muscles to move your spine away from unhealthful positioning into healthy position for daily activities and exercise.

- Puts health back into fitness training. "Fitness" is often unhealthy due to fads, emphasis on cosmetic appearance regardless of toll on joints, lack of information about how muscles really work, and lack of transferring healthy movement skills to everyday life.

How to Use Ab Revolution for Squats

If you exercise for health, with or without weights, neutral spine for squatting increases abdominal muscle use, and is healthier overall exercise, than squatting with hyperlordosis. When using neutral spine properly, you will feel weight shift from your lower spine to core muscles. You will still get good exercise for back muscles, but no longer compress, wear, and degenerate the joints and discs.

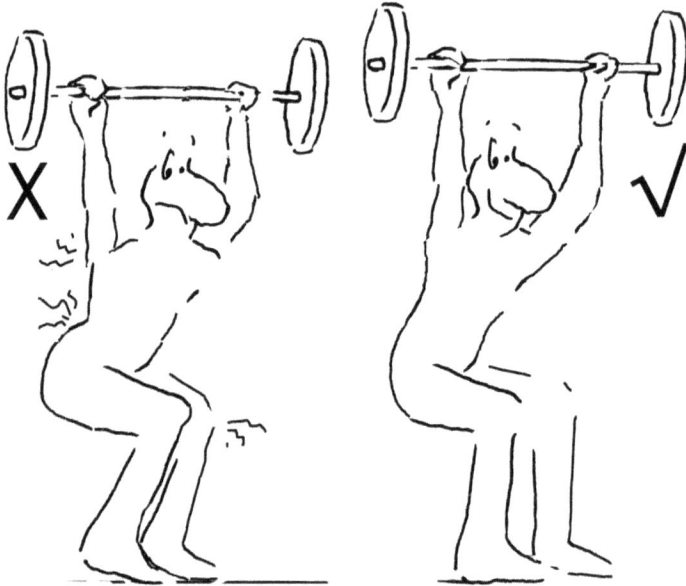

Left: Hyperdordosis during lifts pinches and deforms the lower spine under the combined weight of the upper body plus the load lifted.
Right: Neutral spine. Healthier and more exercise.

Swayback for squats became popularized, even though not healthy. The too-large lumbar curve of hyperlordosis seems to "work" since you can lift more. Hyperlordosis shifts some of the weight and stabilization work off your core muscles and onto the lower spine joints and soft tissue. Muscles work less, so the lift seems easier. Some people believe they are better or stronger by lifting more. The muscles are not getting the intended strengthening. The lower spine is getting extra wear from unhealthy compression.

There are people who deliberately overly increase spinal angle to hyperlordosis, thinking that the resulting unhealthful large lumbar arch is a positive look, similar to believing that smoking a cigarette looks positive, rather than generally unhealthy. There are exercise programs that teach to tilt the pelvis forward, push the backside far to the back, and increase lumbar sway. The reason for that fad seems to have come from thinking it would avoid or correct the opposite problem of rounding the spine. However, overcompensating so that the lower spine overly curves inward is also unhealthful.

If you aren't sure how to move your spine to neutral position for squats, use the Part I section, "A Few Ways to Fix Hyperlordosis and Learn Neutral Spine."

Check and correct knee positioning. A separate problem during squatting affects the knee. Check if you shift body weight forward so that the knees come forward or heels lift from the floor. Effort shifts off the thigh and hip muscles and onto the knee joint. This is common when Achilles tendons are tight. Keep heels down on the floor and knees over heels (right-hand drawing of squat, previous page). You get free, built-in, Achilles tendon stretch every time you bend right, and you will shift weight from knee joints to leg muscles where it belongs.

How to Use Ab Revolution When Lifting Overhead

When lifting weights, leaning the upper body backward or tilting the hip forward shifts load off abdominal muscles and onto lower spine joints, making the lift feel easier. To lift extreme weight and for emergencies, using assists which increase lumbar sway may be the only way to get the weight lifted, even if it is not good for the spine joints over long term use. When lifting for exercise and health, neutral spine is healthier for the spine and gives more exercise for the lifting muscles.

Add balance and stability
Stand on one foot using neutral spine when lifting weights to add balance, strength, and stabilization training for the whole body.

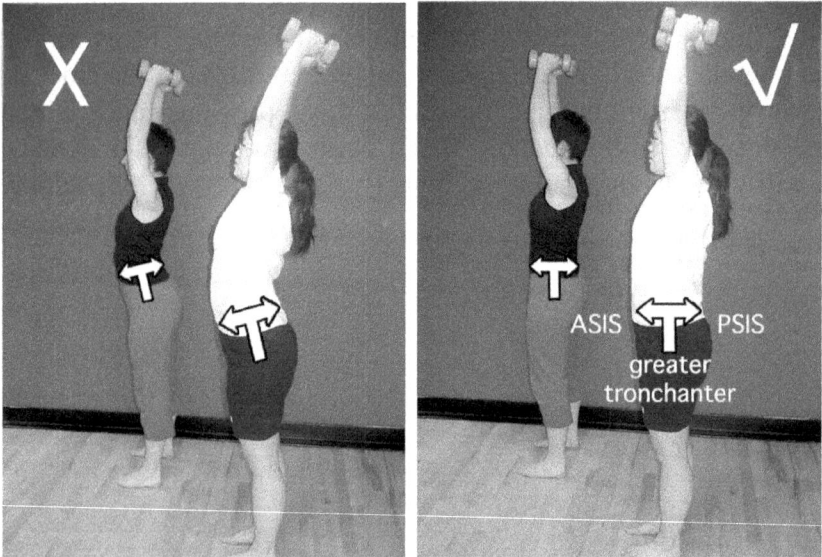

Left: Can you identify the downward tilted belt line, upward rib line, thoracic lean-back, and shortened lumbar length? Right: Same lift using abdominal muscles to reduce hyperlordosis to neutral spine. Belt line is level. Upper body is vertical. Lumbar muscles lengthened for built-in stretch. More exercise for arms and abdominal muscles. Healthier for spine.

Putting Squat and Overhead Lift Together in One Continuous Exercise

---

The previous two sections covered neutral spine for healthier, more effective, squatting and overhead lifting.

This drill practices continuous movement alternating squatting down to pick up weight(s) from the floor, rise and lift overhead, squat to touch the weights to the floor, rise and lift overhead again, repeatedly, smoothly, all using neutral spine, and healthy knee and neck positioning.

1. Choose two hand weights that you can safely lift, or one barbell or other weight that you have practiced with.

2. Choose a number of times you wish to try this, for example ten times to start, or if you are working to eight-count music, then how many sets of eight you want to do.

3. Keep neutral spine for each squat downward. Don't increase lumbar inward curve or outward rounding.

4. Keep neutral spine for each lift overhead; keep pelvis vertical and upper body upright and vertical, not leaning backward. Keep both heels down on the floor throughout the squat.

5. Move in continuous smooth manner, breathing easily. Train to use this for real life situations needing retrieving objects from the ground and lifting them to various heights overhead in neutral spine.

Using Ab Revolution To Fix Triceps Curls

Notice if you allow hyperlordosis for overhead curls. The lower spine joints bear the weight instead of core and arm muscles. You diminish arm exercise, plus miss the abdominal workout you would get if you used abdominal muscles to maintain neutral spine.

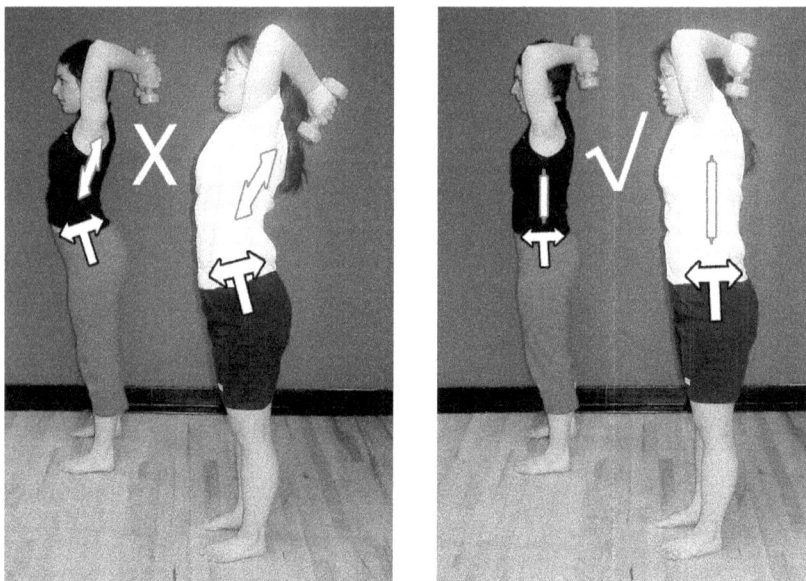

Left: Hyperlordosis: Anterior hip tilt. Beltline tips down in front. Side seam from middle hip crest to the top of the leg tilts forward. Upper body leans backward. Shortened lumbar length. Right: Same lift using abs to reduce hyperlordosis to neutral.

1. If the pelvis is tilted, tuck the pelvis to make the line vertical from the side of the hip down to top of the leg bone.
2. If you lean the upper body backward, pull forward until vertical and straight.

By returning to neutral spine, you shift the weight of your upper body, plus the weights, off your lower spine. You will feel effort shift to your core muscles.

Using Ab Revolution To Fix Lunges and Warrior Pose

Yoga won't automatically "give" you good posture. You must consciously move your body out of injurious position and into healthy position when practicing poses.

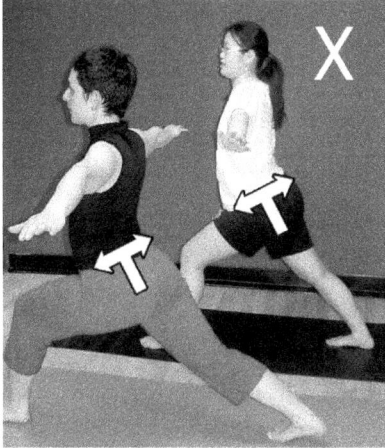

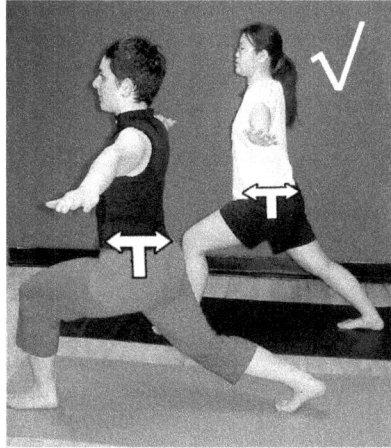

Left: Hyperlordosis. Belt line tips downward in front. Side seam tilts forward. Lumbar and anterior hip muscle length shortened. Right: Same pose with abdominals in use to reduce hyperlordosis to neutral spine. Belt line level. Pelvis vertical. Lumbar compression stopped. More stretch in hip and leg.

1. Use abdominal muscles to tuck pelvis to vertical, bring upper body vertical, and reduce lumbar overarch to neutral.
2. Feel increase in abdominal use, and no more lower spine compression.
3. Done correctly, you will feel better leg and anterior hip stretch.

Some styles of yoga teach to deliberately cause hyperlordosis for many poses. Letting the spine sag into hyperlordosis does not use abdominal muscles and is an ironic contributor to back and hip pain for those doing yoga believing it magically or automatically fixes pain or posture. Use neutral spine for lunges and yoga poses such as warrior.

Special Ab Revolution Exercise – Isometric Abs

Isometric Abs is a fun retraining drill to develop abdominal muscles and practice how to use them to hold healthy spine position against resistance. This drill also improves shoulder range of motion and function when lifting. These are not crunches. Your upper body never lifts from the floor.

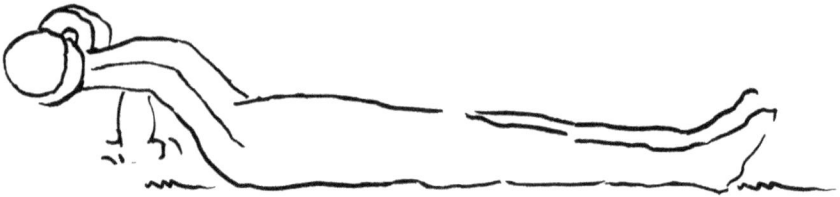

Functional abdominal exercise uses straight legs. Abdominal muscles, not knees, control spine posture and prevent the lumbar spine from increasing in arch and lifting from the floor. The hand weights are lifted only a few inches above the floor.

1. Lie face up, arms on the floor, biceps by your ears. Legs straight.

2. Hold hand weights an inch above the floor. Notice if you allow ribs to lift and lower back to rise from the floor. Instead, press your lower back toward the floor.

3. You will feel your abdominal muscles working to maintain spine position. Done right, there is no pain in lower spine.

4. Breathe normally. Practice using your abdominals to maintain spine position without tightening or restricting breathing.

5. Raise and lower the weights rapidly many times, between one and four or five inches above the floor. As the weight lowers, the momentum and weight may encourage lifting the ribs and arching the back to shift the work of the exercise from the

abdominal muscles to the vertebral joints. Use abdominal muscles to prevent this. Your lower spine never lifts from the floor.

6. Do not raise the upper body or head from the floor. Learn to relax the head and neck. Use the abdominal muscles, without pressing the back of the head or upper body more against the floor to counter the weight.

Your abdominal muscles work hard on this *Isometric Abs* exercise to hold spine positioning against the weight. This drill also works the arms and back while stretching the hip. The benefit is to learn to use abdominal muscles to hold safe, effective, and functional neutral spine posture when using the rest of your body. You get several exercises at once, and practice working your body the way you need for real life movement.

If it is not comfortable to lie flat, the front of your hip may be too tight. Stretching the front of your hip and other specific places can solve discomfort from being too tight to lie comfortably flat. See the end of Part I, which explains what to do "When Your Lower Back Hurts to Lie Flat Without A Pillow."

If your shoulders are too tight to lie flat with arms overhead, you are too tight to stand and reach up without being pulled into hyperlordosis. Use this drill to help stretch the upper body safely.

Use the *Isometric Abs* drill to practice for daily life activities that need standing with healthy spine position and straight legs.

Why Isn't It Necessary To Keep Knees Bent?

It is commonly repeated that knees must be bent "to protect the back" or "keep your back from arching" or "to put your back into proper position" when doing abdominal and core exercise. However, your own abdominal muscles can and should position your spine, which is the point of The Isometric Abs drill. Instead of bending knees, learn to control your spine with legs straight, the same as you need for standing and going about your life.

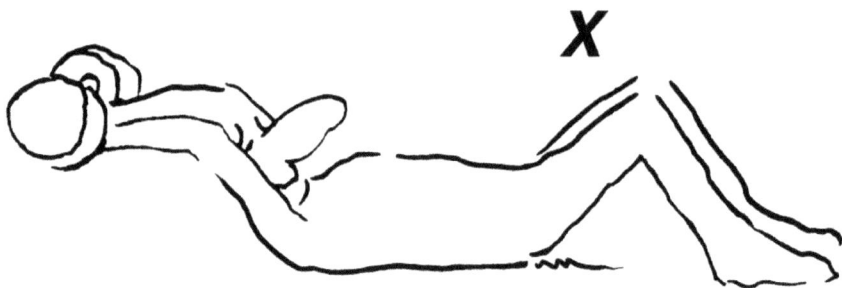

Bent knees reduces abdominal exercise, and does not train abdominal use for standing. Using core muscles to maintain neutral vertebral angle, not bending knees, is what prevents painful angle and load.

By keeping knees bent, you never learn to use your core muscles to reposition the spine from swayback to neutral when standing. If it were true that the way to protect the back is to bend the knees and hip, then how are you supposed to stand and walk home? With knees and hips bent that much too?

Many people keep the hip bent while standing in daily life, then exercise that way. Bending knees feeds a negative cycle of tight anterior hip muscles, bent hip, a spine in overarched painful posture when standing, and, ironically, minimal abdominal muscle use.

Another common instruction is to stand with one foot in front of the other or one foot up on a block to reduce pain. Standing swaybacked causes the pain, not foot placement. You can directly reduce a swayed lumbar spine by moving your spine to neutral using abdominal muscles without needing to raise one foot or bend your knees.

Instead of strange rules about standing in bent ways, use your abdominal muscles to reduce the painfully arched position and return to comfortable neutral spine. Done correctly, discomfort from hyperlordosis in the lower back should be gone. Use Isometric Abs to practice it against resistance.

Carryover to Real Life
Think of all the exercises and daily life activities that involve lifting weight overhead and preventing hyperlordosis, as practiced with the *Isometric Abs* drill. When you do standing weight lifting, and activities around the house like putting away laundry and groceries, remember to control your spine position with what you learned and practice from *Isometric Abs*.

If you aren't sure how to move your spine from swayback to neutral, use the Part I section, "A Few Ways to Fix Hyperlordosis and Learn Neutral Spine."

Ab Revolution Neutral Spine Planks

Pushups and planks (holding a pushup position) are often cited as core muscle exercise. However, when they are done in hyperlordosis, the abdominals do not get the intended exercise. Body weight rests on the vertebrae, not core muscles. Letting the lower back sag into an arch is a missed opportunity to strengthen your muscles, and is hard on the spine joints and soft tissue. Keep spine neutral and you will train core strength and stability, and upper and lower body strength.

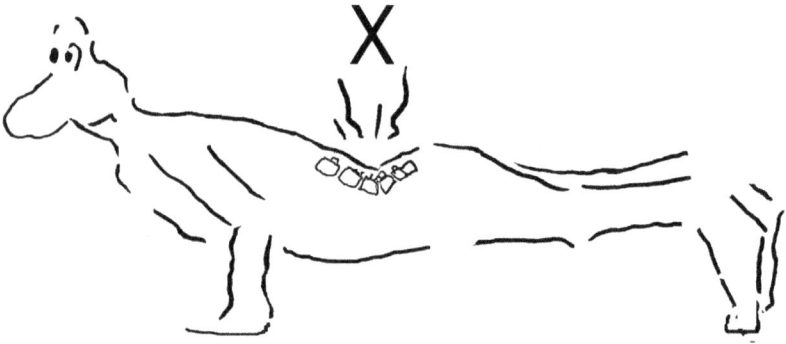

Hyperlordosis. Lower back folding into painful increased arch.

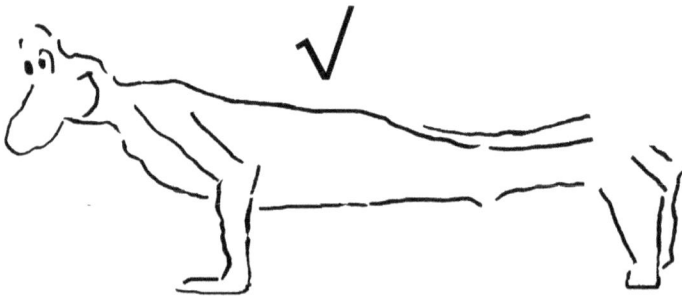

Neutral spine. Done right, you will immediately feel abdominal muscles in use, and pain disappears from the lower spine.

Holding the pushup position (plank)

1. Hold the high pushup position (plank). Tuck the pelvis under to straighten the spine, as if starting a lower body crunch motion. Feel immediate shift of the work to abdominals.

2. Don't sag your spine or lift your hip and backside upward to make it easier. Allowing hyperlordosis is not modifying an exercise, but circumventing it.

3. Hold your head in line with your body. The phrase, "Be straight as a plank" includes the entire spine.

4. Keep elbows slightly bent. Don't lock them straight. If your arms are too weak to hold you, you need to strengthen them, not add wear to your elbow joints.

5. Keep your weight on your entire hand not only the heel, to prevent compression of the wrist joints. Vary hand positioning to strengthen hands. Planks/pushups on fists is shown below.

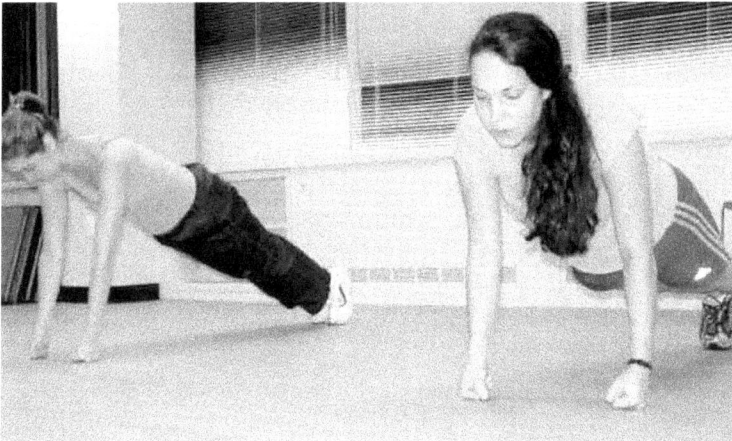

For challenge and fun, put hands on a balance board, ball, roller, cushion, or other wobbly object for safe, higher training. Then try holding flat stable neutral plank lifting one hand, then the other, keeping body flat, not tilted or turned, shown in next section.

Try fun real life games using the plank

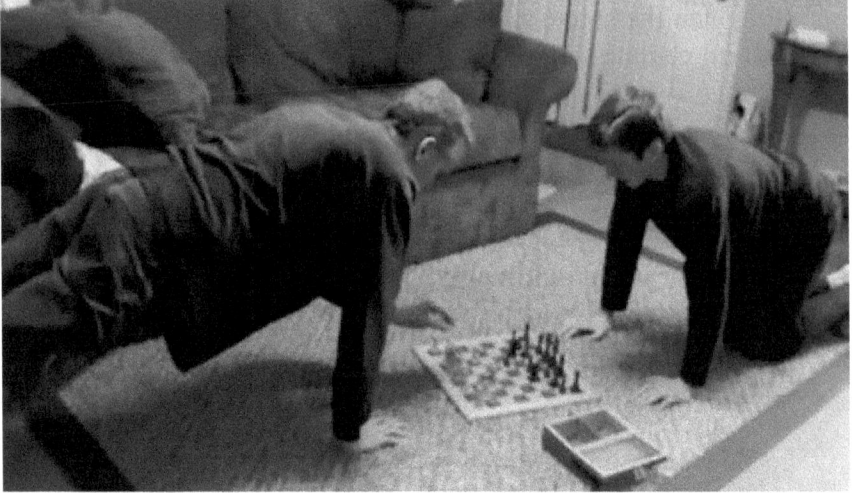

If you cannot hold up your own body weight without slouching after mere seconds, how able are you to hold healthy position all day during real life? Practice to increase the time you can hold your posture without sagging. If you lift weights to strengthen your back, remember that the most important weight to be able to lift is your own body, in healthful position.

In addition to getting good exercise, use knowledge of how to hold a push up position without increasing lumbar sway to train and practice neutral spine to use when standing.

If you aren't sure how to stop hyperlordosis and move your spine to neutral, use the Part I section, "A Few Ways to Fix Hyperlordosis and Learn Neutral Spine."

Ab Revolution Planks Lifting Arms and Legs

1. Hold a neutral spine plank (previous section). Lift one leg, maintaining neutral spine.

2. Add lifting the opposite arm, with neutral spine (or just past neutral to flat), not allowing increase in lumbar arch.

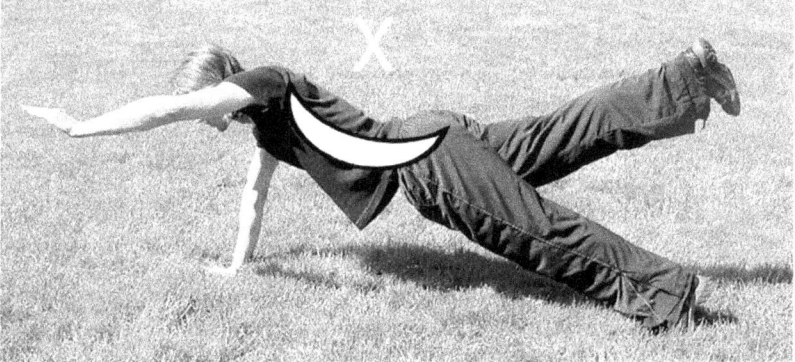

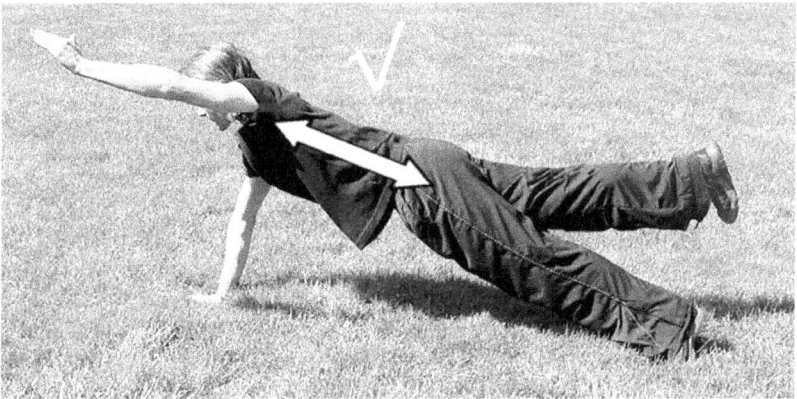

Top: Hyperlordosis. Weight sags onto spine soft tissue and spine joints called facets. Bottom: Neutral spine. Leg lifted with hip and leg muscles, not by changing spine angle. Arm and head level with body.

Notice if you sway your spine to lift your arm or leg. Instead, reduce the large curve of hyperlordosis when you lift your limbs. When you do this correctly, you will immediately feel high abdominal exercise, and spine compression from hyperlordosis will stop.

Don't turn or lift your body to the side. Stay level.

For challenge and fun, place one hand or one foot (or both) on a balance board, ball, roller, cushion, or other wobbly object for safe, higher training, while lifting the other hand and foot, keeping body flat, not tilted or turned.

If you aren't sure how to move to neutral, use the Part I section, "A Few Ways to Fix Hyperlordosis and Learn Neutral Spine."

Ab Revolution Pushups With Neutral Spine

Allowing the spine to sag in hyperlordosis makes pushups feel easier to do because the abdominal muscles don't have to work. The weight of the body which should be held on the abdominals rests instead on the spine joints called facets. Surrounding soft issue is pinched and uncomfortably folded backwards. If you are exercising for health and exercise, then get the exercise by using neutral spine. Notice hyperlordosis in three of the four people doing pushups, pictured below:

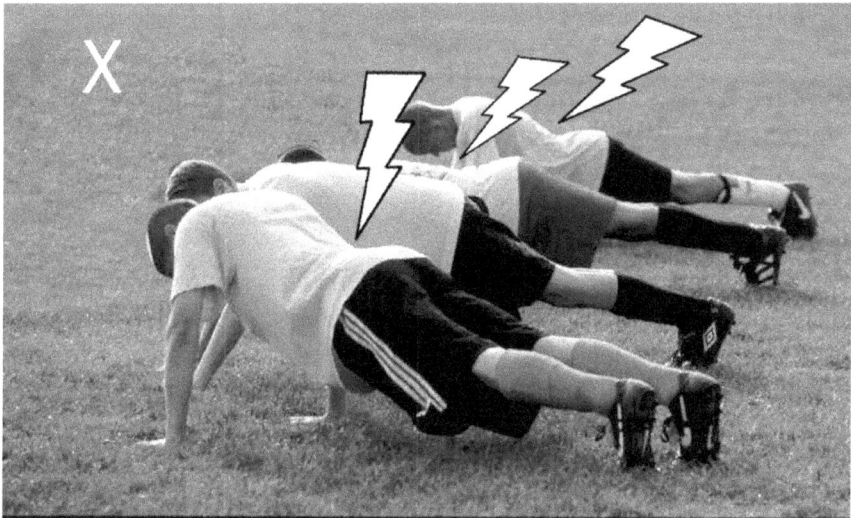

Hyperlordosis (first, third, and last on right). Abdominal muscles not in use. Weight of the body "hammocks" onto lower back joints and soft tissue. Second from left is neutral, although head and neck slouch downward.

1. Check during pushups if you let your spine sag. Tuck pelvis under to neutral spine, or just past it to flat. Don't round your back or lift your hip and backside in the air.

2. Done correctly, you will feel the pushup change into an abdominal and core exercise.

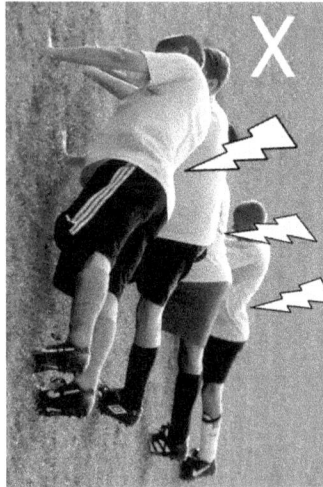

Turning the previous image sideways shows how the first, third, and fourth person would look standing – unhealthy lumbar sway, head hanging, and lack of use of abdominal and other muscles.

Even if you can't do pushups, try. Hold a neutral spine pushup position (plank) on hands and feet, not hands and knees, and do small dips and raises. Add more each week. It is a quick, effective exercise for most of your body, including the important weak link of wrists and hands.

"Reverse" pushups
For "reverse" pushups where you lie on the floor first and push upward to a straight arm position, don't allow your upper body to rise first, which increases lumbar angle. Stay flat and rise as a unit.

Transfer neutral spine pushup practice to standing during daily activities
Remember to transfer the knowledge of using abdominals during exercise, to change spine posture during real life when standing and moving.

Ab Revolution Plank Rows

Hold the plank to lift weights:

1. Hold a neutral spine pushup position.

2. Lift a weight from the floor to your chest with one hand (like rowing). Keep body flat, not tilted to one side. Don't allow the spine to sag downward or lift upward at any point.

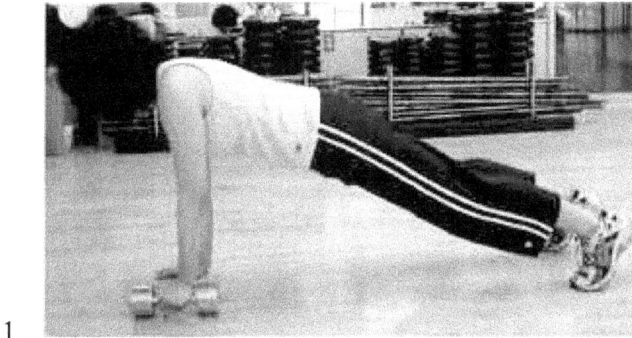

1.

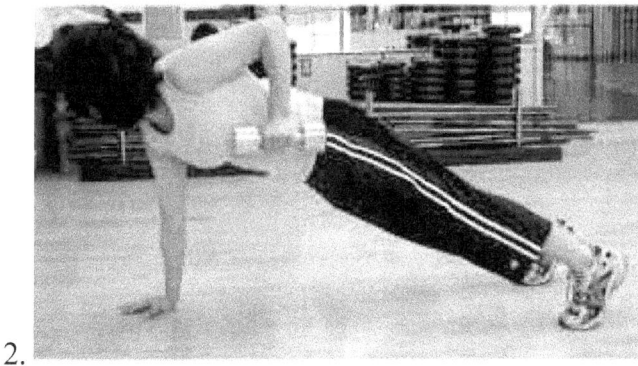

2.

Use different arm exercises while in the plank. Try curls, flies, straight arm, and other variations of lifts. For challenge and fun, put one hand on a balance board, ball, foam roller, cushion, or other wobbly object for safe, higher training. Add holding one leg off the floor.

Ab Revolution High Planks With Neutral Spine - Handstand

Neutral spine high plank can be fun and safe, done with care and awareness. It is not as hard as it looks.

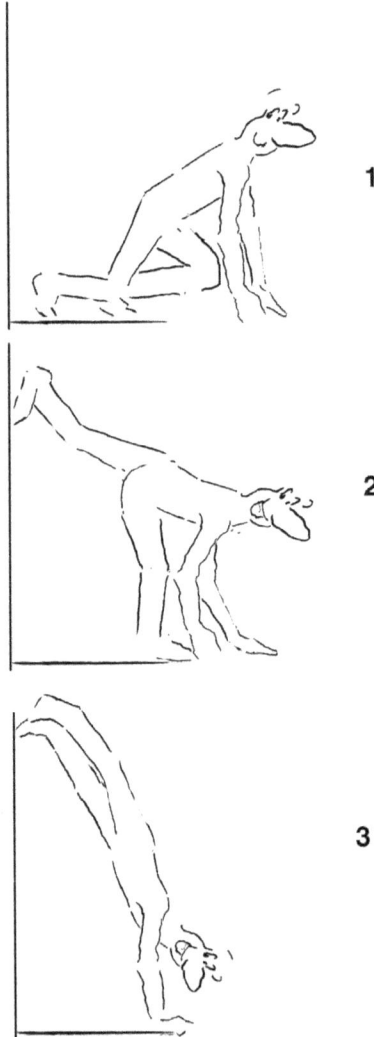

1. Stand about three feet from a wall with your back to the wall. Crouch down. Put both hands on the floor.

2. Put the bottom of one foot high up on the wall behind you. Lift the other foot.

3. Check lumbar spine position and move to neutral if needed. Hold your body straight.

Make sure to prevent hyperlordosis during handstand / high planks. The handstand is a great opportunity to train neutral spine. See the photo below for what to look for.

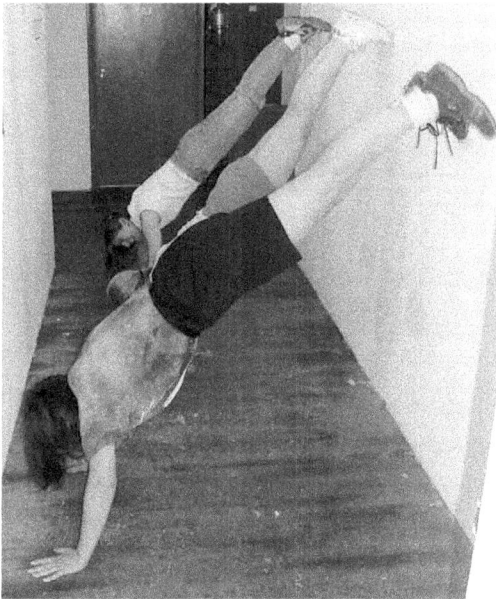

First from left (closest figure) is holding hip bent and hiked upward
Second and third are straighter and more neutral at spine and hip.

To get started
If you need to get confidence first, do a plank with your feet up on a low bench. Then try a higher chair or ledge. Use a low ledge to work abs more, and a higher one to work arms more. Notice and correct spine position from any sway.

High Plank or Wall Handstand With Rows

To increase abilities, balance, strength, and more:

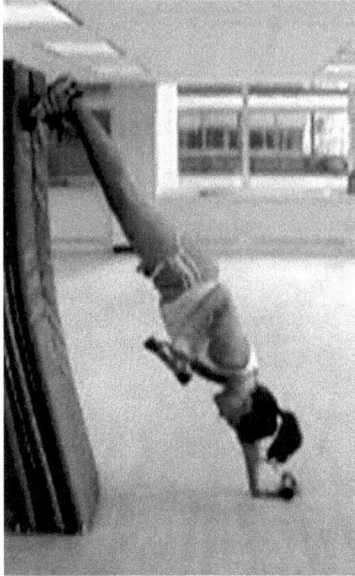

1. Once you learned the neutral spine high plank handstand described previously, practice shifting weight from hand to hand until you can stand on one hand alone.

2. Lift a hand weight with the other hand for upside down rows.

3. Hold the handstand and bend arms for small dips, to do upside-down presses. Work to increase the distance you can safely dip and the number of times.

4. To work for better balance, reduce your need for the wall and increasingly learn to balance in handstand without it.

The wrist and upper spine are two of three main sites of osteoporosis. Handstands of all kinds help increase bone density in arms, wrists, and upper spine, helpful for osteoporosis prevention.

Wheelbarrows

The wheelbarrow can be a fun partner exercise.

1. The first partner holds a plank, not allowing the lower back to sag. The second partner picks up the first partner's legs at the ankles.

2. The second partner walks forward and to the sides in any direction holding the first partner's ankles. The first partner must walk on hands, maintaining neutral spine using abs at all times against all the variations in resistance and directions.

Group wheelbarrows can be done with both partners in plank and the first partner's feet on the second's shoulders. Add a third partner to lift the second's legs. Be safe and creative. Have fun.

Increase Weight To Increase Strength While Holding Neutral Position

Add a weight during pushups. If you use neutral spine, increased resistance adds postural challenge and safely increases strength and endurance over time of those muscles and ability.

Start with a knapsack or other light weight. Increase safely. Don't let your lower back sag under the weight. Use this exercise to learn to keep your back safer.

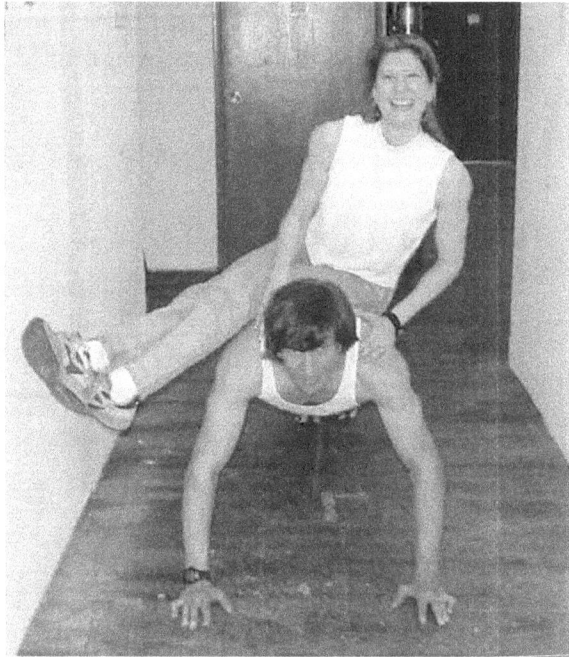

Adding extra weight can be done safely if you use more effort in abdominal and core muscles to keep back and body in healthy position.

Walking And Jumping Pushups (Spiders)

To increase strength, balance, power, and spine position control, try these fun, effective, walking and jumping planks:

- Hold a neutral spine plank. Keep your head and neck in line with your body. Maintain the same spine posture you would want if you were standing up.

- "Walk" your arms and legs to move around like a flat spider. Walk sideways, forward, backward, and randomly. Move quickly and slowly.

- Keeping neutral pushup position, jump like a flat jumping spider. Don't allow your back to sag under the momentum of landing. Use good shock absorption with arms and legs.

- Make several jumps sideways across the room. Jump to the next piece of furniture or exercise equipment. Jump to say hello to someone.

- Jump 90 degrees with each jump to face each direction. Start facing front, then jump to the left, back, right, then front again. Then jump four times back the other way–from front to right, back, left, to the front again. Have fun. Work up to full half turns, eventually to full 360 jumps.

"Spiders" effectively work arm and leg muscles, and the core if you use muscles to maintain neutral spine posture. They are effective and safe if you protect your back with healthy spine positioning and shock absorption.

If you aren't sure how to move to neutral spine, use the Part I section, "A Few Ways to Fix Hyperlordosis and Learn Neutral Spine."

The Flag

Holding the body straight without support for the feet is sometimes called "The Flag." Use the flag to train neutral spine under high resistance, then transfer that strength and knowledge to other high resistance activities of all kinds. Experiment with varied leg placement. This move can be done safely or not, well or not. The idea of The Ab Revolution is to involve thinking to use healthy positioning, not only for the moment, but to other activities in life.

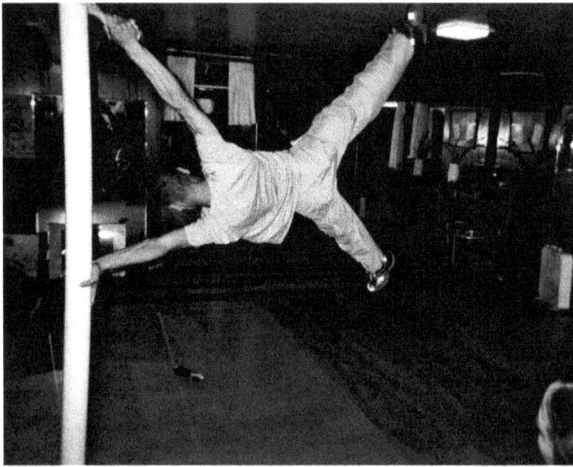

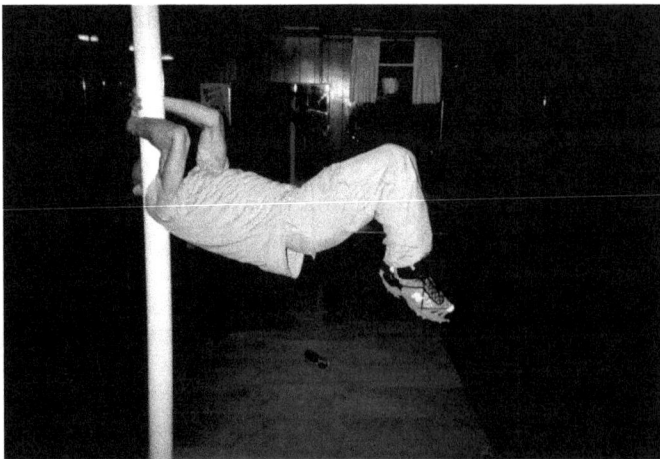

Using Oblique Abs to Control Spine—Side Arm Planks

Use side planks to consciously train straight torso positioning to transfer to use when standing. You will exercise the oblique abdominal muscles, and help bone density of the wrist, if you stand on the hand, not elbow.

1. Hold the pushup position and turn to one side. Lift one arm and balance on the other arm.

2. Hold your body straight. Don't sag or lift the hip.

3. Keep your elbow slightly bent. Don't lock it straight. Save your elbow joint and get an arm workout.

4. Keep your weight on your entire hand, not concentrated on the heel, to prevent compressing the wrist. Hold as long as you can then switch sides and repeat.

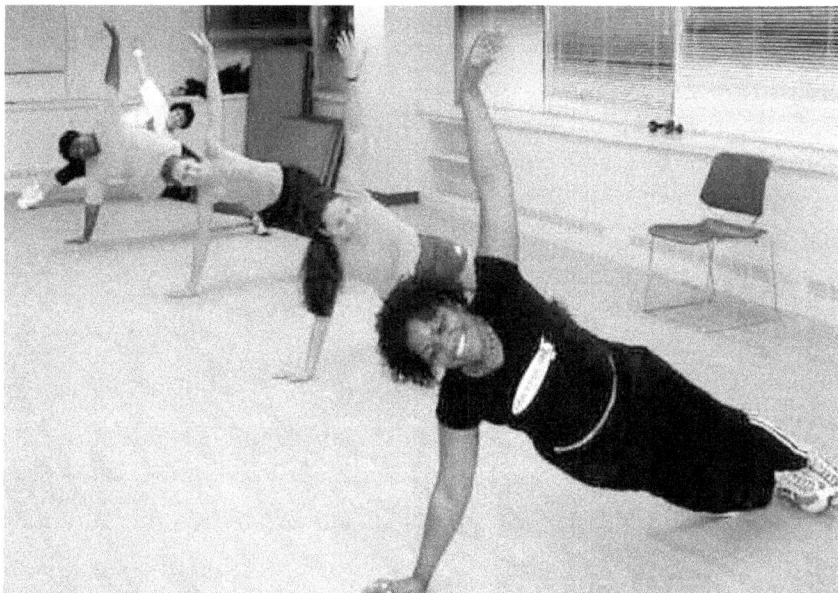

- In the side position, raise your top leg and hold to stretch the leg. Then raise and lower your top leg from the floor as many times as you can, maintaining straight torso posture.

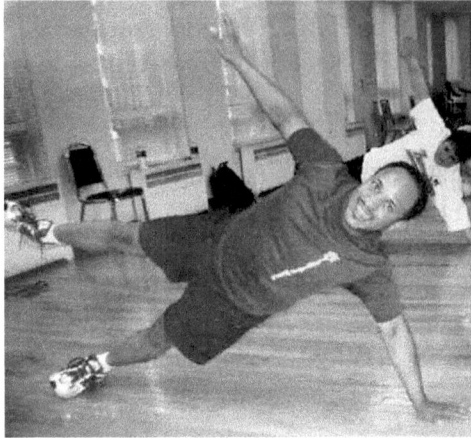

- For variation, move the top leg forward and hold it out in front as long as you can. Then try stretching the raised leg behind you, both with straight leg, and bending the knee for front hip and thigh stretch.

Benefit to wrists

The wrist and upper spine are two of three major sites of osteoporosis. Weight bearing exercise improves arm and spine bone density and strength, two more benefits of Ab Revolution exercises. To prevent wrist pain, keep your weight distributed on your entire hand not only the heel of the hand. Press forward with the muscles of your hands and fingers, to offset compression of the wrist backward.

Check when you type, drive, prepare food, and during other daily activities, that you do not compress wrists backward under the resistance of your activity. There is no need to hold wrists straight or splint them. Movement is crucial for all joint health. Use hand strength when using your hands, don't let the weight compress or twist the joints. Using hand and arm muscles will also strengthen hands and wrists so that your wrists better able to work during everyday activity.

More Challenging Ab Revolution Moves for Oblique Abdominal Muscles

1. Hold a pushup position. Lift one leg 90 degrees to the side, as if swinging it over a bicycle. You will get enough range of motion of the leg if you rotate toes and knees to face forward, not downward. Keep your leg straight and parallel to the floor, not tilting downward. Sometimes this exercise is called "The Peeing Dog" for the position of the leg straight out to the side.

2. Keep a strong hip tuck to prevent your spine from sagging. Keep your body flat, not turned to the side. Don't lift or tilt your hips or backside upward. Hold flat position as long as you can, then switch legs.

3. Try pushups while holding the leg straight out to the side.

4. To advance, add lifting the opposite arm.

5. Work up to switching sides by jumping from leg to leg, rather than putting one down before lifting the other. During each landing, prevent the lumbar spine from arching.

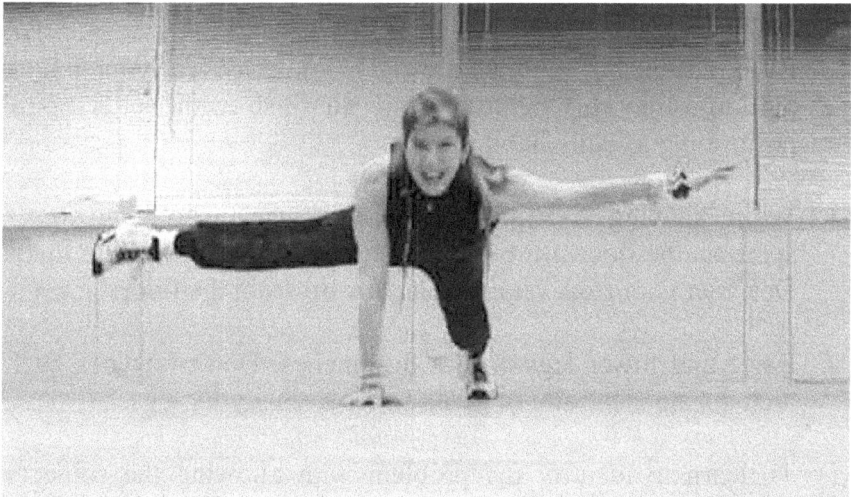

Use Abs, Not Hands, to Reposition the Spine For Leg Lifts

Front leg lifts primarily use leg and hip muscles that bend your leg at the hip, called hip flexors, not abdominal muscles. Where abdominal muscles are needed is to prevent the lower back from increasing in arch to counter the weight of the lifted legs. You need to add this abdominal action deliberately. It does not come from leg lifts alone.

Do you need leg lifts to the front?
Most people do not need to practice more bending at the hip. They are already too tight and bent. Tight short hip flexors reduce ability to stand, lie down, or move in healthy ways.

How to change leg lifts to use abdominals
If you have special athletic activities that need more hip flexor strength, like martial arts, ballet, or climbing, and you use leg lifts to improve those, then you need to know how to use abdominal muscles to prevent hyperlordosis when lifting the legs. It is better for your back, and you get more and healthier abdominal exercise.

1. Lie on your back with legs straight and flat on the floor. Press your lower back against the floor and feel your abdominals work to do this. Feel the change in spine and hip tilt.

2. If your front hip muscles are tight, you may feel your thighs pull upward. Hip tightness will diminish with better spine positioning as daily habit.

3. While keeping abdominal muscles in use to hold the lower spine on the floor, lift both legs an inch or two above the floor. Don't let your back return to arch or lift from the floor.

4. Raise and lower legs only a few inches. Don't let your back arch during any point of raising or lowering your legs.

5. To learn to identify the problem with allowing the spine to arch, let your lumbar spine increase the arch and lift high from the floor. Lift your legs an inch or two above the floor. You

may feel the weight of your legs pinching your lower back. Don't do this if you have back pain. Use for education and understanding Doing leg lifts this way is not good for you, and does not use abdominal muscles.

6. Return your lower back position to the floor and repeat the lift. Done correctly, you should feel back pain from arching disappear, and a good amount of effort shift to your abdominal muscles.

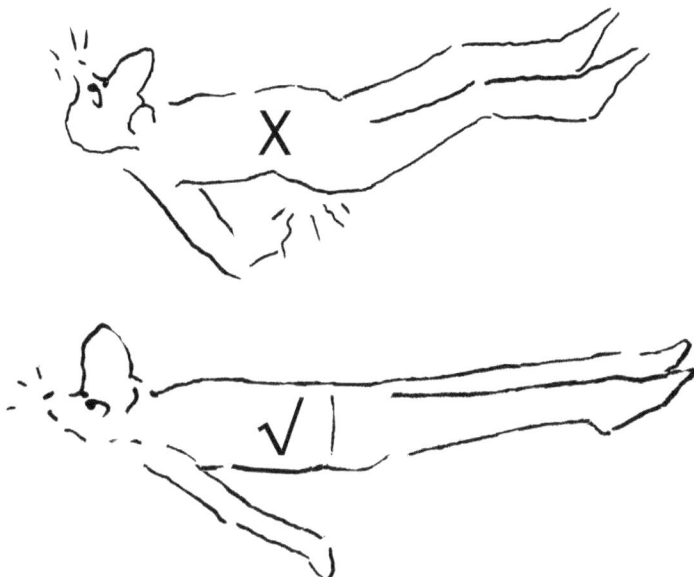

Leg lifts may sometimes be taught with the instruction that hands under the hip "keep the back from arching." However, using hands prevents you from using your own abdominal muscles to do that. If you aren't sure how to move to neutral, use the Part I section, "A Few Ways to Fix Hyperlordosis and Learn Neutral Spine."

Remember that front leg lifts are not a functional or needed exercise for most people. Hip flexors do not need more training to bend forward. If you want strong core exercise, use the effective, functional exercises throughout this book.

Back Leg Lifts

The best exercise for back muscles is exercise that uses them to practice neutral spine during movement used in real life activity.

Many common exercises don't train back muscles as needed for real movement or healthy spine positioning. One example is bending over to lift weights. It may work muscles, but sheers and unequally bulges discs over time. This is why bending over is not healthy to pick up packages. Instead of bending over to lift weights, use Neutral Spine Squats for healthy bending, and Ab Revolution Plank Rows for back strengthening, both shown earlier in Part II.

Another conventional back exercise is back leg lifts on hands and knees, sometimes called "bird-dog." Watch for the mistake of arching the spine to lift the leg, instead of lifting with hip and leg muscles in neutral spine.

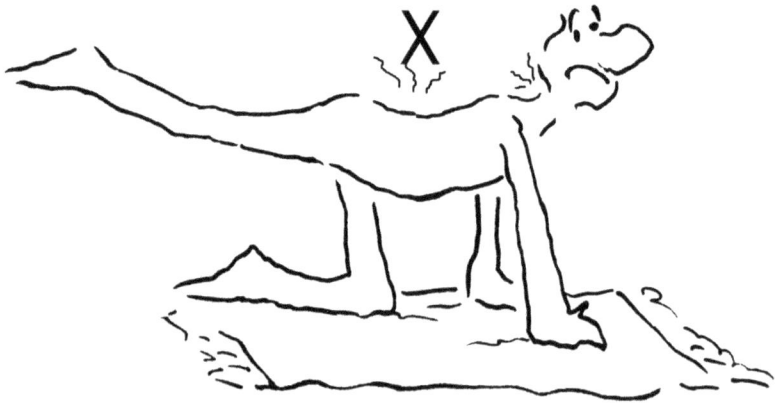

Arching the spine reduces involvement of leg and back muscles, compresses lower spine joints, and reinforces faulty movement patterns—to move your leg by arching your back. Watch for the same injurious body mechanics of arching when walking and running, instead of maintaining neutral spine with abdominals, and using muscles of the leg and posterior hip to extend the leg.

Try the following to feel how to use abdominal, hip, and leg muscles, not spine, to lift your leg:

1. Notice if you arch your spine to lift your leg. Tuck your hip under to bring your back to a straight position. If you are not sure how, see Part I.

2. Use leg, hip, and gluteal muscles to lift your leg instead of bending from the spine. You will feel immediate shift of work to your abdomen, and far more exercise for your back, hip, and leg.

3. Use upper back muscles to hold head and neck in line with your back. Keep chin level, not lifted, which bends the neck back at unhealthy angle. Lift from your chest to look forward without craning your neck.

You may find you cannot lift your leg as high. That is because you were previously lifting your leg by arching your back, pivoting on the spine joints. Instead, get real leg exercise, while getting built-in abdominal exercise.

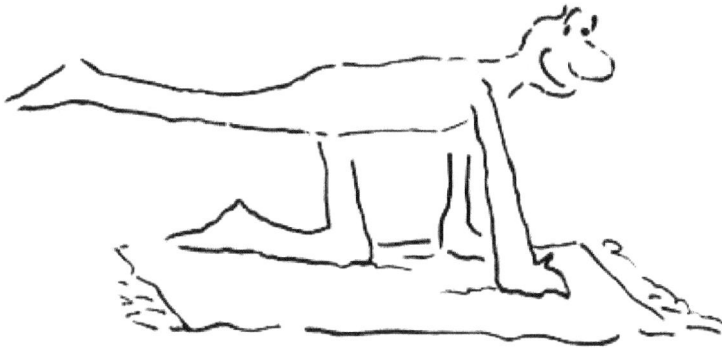

You can use this hands and knees position to quickly learn neutral spine, but it is so little exercise that it is far better to get off the knees and hold a simple plank, shown next.

Next, get off your knees. "Hands and knees position" gives little exercise and does not train you how to hold your body position against gravity.

1. Hold a real pushup position. It will strengthen your arms and body in a better, functional way. Use abdominal muscles to tuck your hip to straighten your spine, or you will get little core exercise.

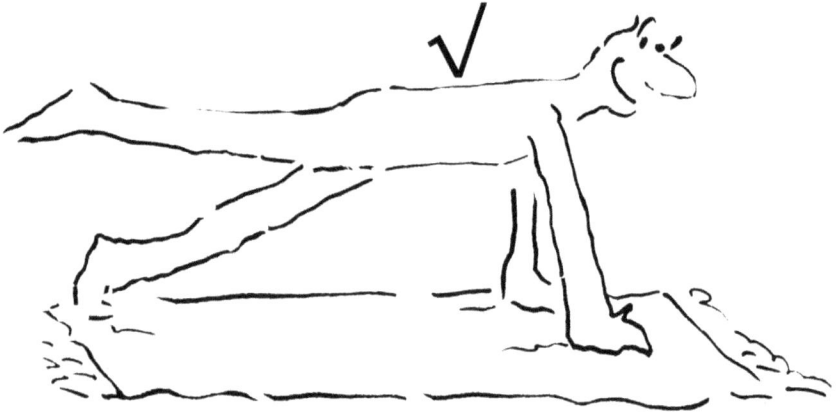

2. Lift one leg, holding healthy straight body position.

3. When you can hold a straight plank with one leg up, lift the opposite arm straight in front also. Don't drop your head. Use muscles to hold you as straight as if you were standing.

Use this neutral spine method to get effective abdominal exercise, and at the same time, retrain to prevent hyperlordosis when you extend legs in back to walk. Transfer the knowledge of how to use good positioning from this drill to all your daily activities when standing and moving.

Using Ab Revolution for Chin-ups and Pull-ups

Regardless of hand position (facing front or back), don't allow your lower back to increase in arch as you pull up and lower. Instead, use abdominal muscles to reduce lumbar curve to neutral.

Retrain the bad habit of practicing poor position of bent hip, ribs lifted, and swayback. Holding straight position increases abdominal muscle use while you practice their function of holding the spine in healthy position. Keep body straight while raising and lowering unless you are practicing for a specific need, for example, climbing or gymnastic moves.

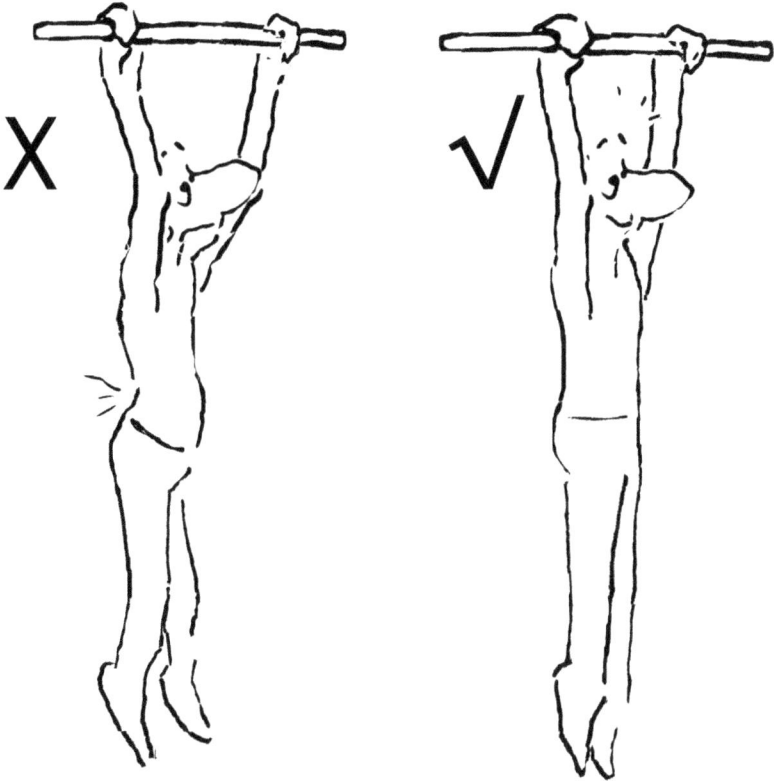

Using Ab Revolution for Pull-Downs

Besides producing one kind of back pain, hyperlordosis reduces effectiveness of many exercises. See for yourself. Try the "pull-down" exercise with healthy spine position. Done right, using abdominal muscles to prevent hyperlordosis, you will feel far more core and arm exercise.

1. Reduce large lumbar curve to neutral.
2. Tuck pelvis to vertical
3. Bring upper body to upright without leaning backward.
4. Then when you are no longer using swayback to assist the exercise, pull the weight down, maintaining neutral spine without leaning back to assist.
5. Add by pulling the bar all the way down to your legs.

To add balance and stability, balance on one foot while pulling down. Maintain neutral spine.

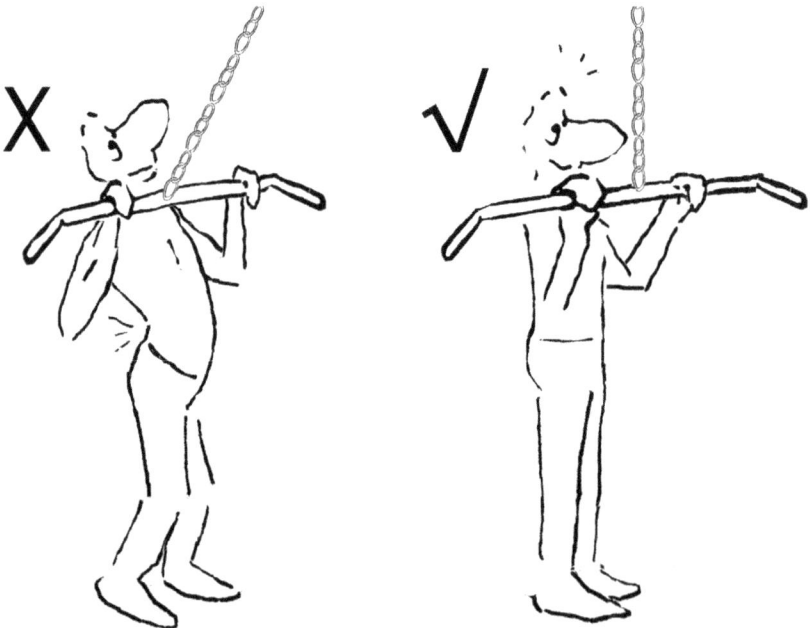

Using Ab Revolution for Handstands and Headstands

Use abdominal muscles to prevent your spine from arching during headstands and handstands.

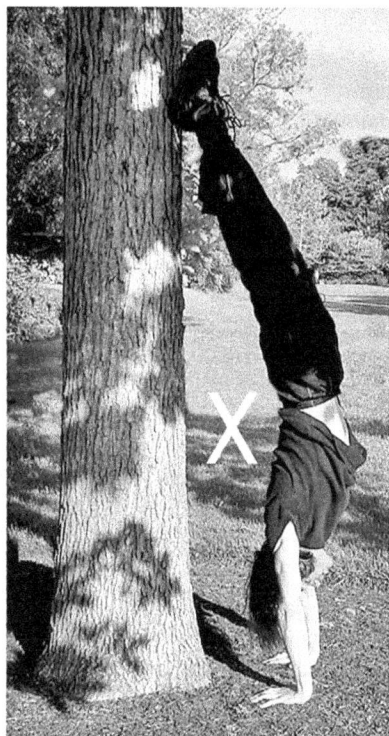

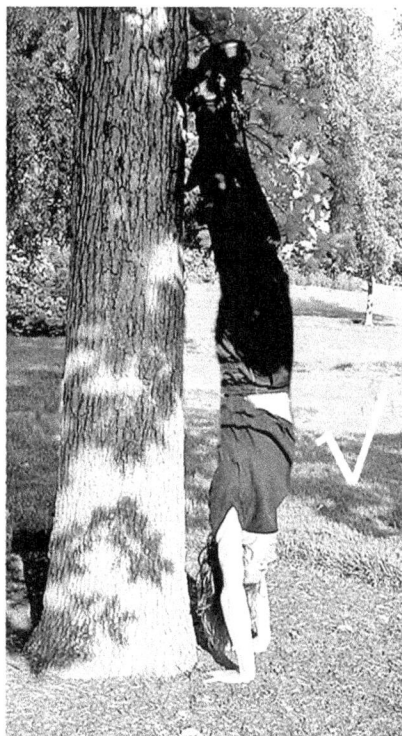

Left: Allowing swayback, compressing the lower spine under the weight of the legs. Right: Reducing arch to reduce lower spine compression, and increase abdominal work.

Straighter position requires more muscle control for balance. Some people prefer to arch because it is easier. Practice straight position for better abdominal strength, to stop spine compression, and improve balance training. Learning supported extension for various extended spine handstand forms and ranges of motion is covered later in Part II.

Ab Revolution Bands and Cables

Maintain neutral spine when using cable pulleys or bands. Allowing hyperlordosis makes the exercise easier because abdominal muscles do not work to hold spine position. You will get more abdominal exercise maintaining neutral spine against resistance.

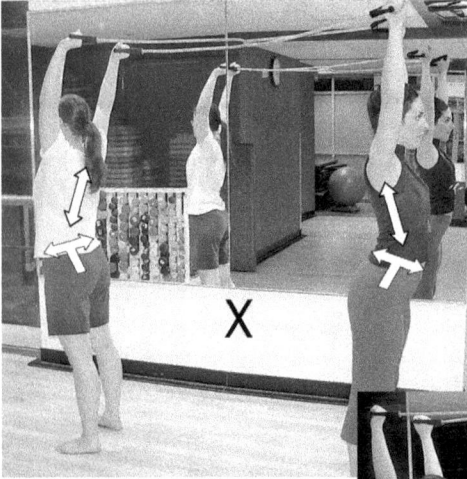

Photograph at left: Both figures demonstrate hyperlordosis. Upper body leans backward.
Hip tilted forward.
Spine compressed.
Abs not in use.

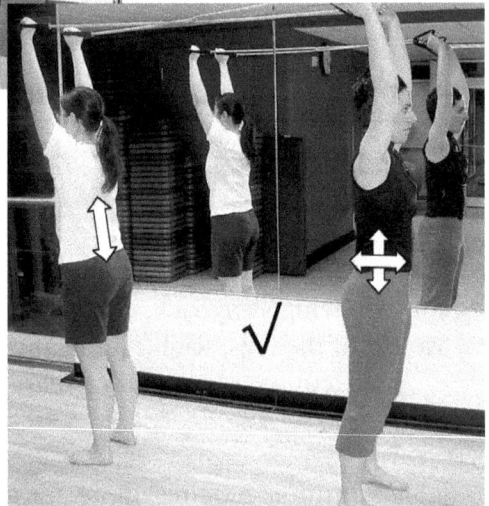

Photograph at right:
Using abdominal muscles to straighten spine to neutral and increase abdominal exercise

To make best use of bands and cable pulls, use arm motions that simulate your sport (pitching, rowing, basketball, throwing, and so on) or activities like washing hair, all while maintaining neutral spine.

Ab Revolution Bands and Cables for Oblique Abdominal Training

Use the following drills to train oblique (side) abdominal muscles to hold spine position against resistance. You will strengthens your oblique abdominal muscles while practicing how to hold your spine from slouching to the side against overhead loads and moving loads.

Using bands and pulleys
1. Use a stretchy band, tubing, pulleys, or even a pair of stretch pants to get started. Secure the middle at about shoulder height. Hold both ends and turn sideways.

2. Move farther away if more tension is wanted on the band.

3. Maintain straight neutral spine posture against the sideways pull of the band. Don't let the band pull you into a sideways bent posture. Stabilize and straighten your body using your oblique abs.

4. Try different arm motions, ranges, exercises, and simulations of needed reaching activities. Keep your torso straight, not twisting from your waist.

5. To progress, hold both arms overhead against your ears, and repeat this exercise, maintaining neutral spine against the pull of the band.

Oblique abdominal practice turning at angles
- Hold the band at a strong tension and face various angles toward and away from the band. Practice moving your arms for common activities, retraining yourself to use abs first, before moving your arms. Try the motion of combing your hair (or washing your head if you're bald), brushing teeth, hanging up clothes, writing on the board, underhand and side pitches, and anything else you need for daily life.

- For each activity, instead of starting the move with only your shoulder and arm, move your spine into neutral position and feel the increase in use of the abdominal muscles first. Then, use the power of the torso (core) muscles to turn your body and power the arm movement.

Moving stabilization drills
- Walk around, side to side, and diagonally, keeping your body upright against the changing pull of the band.

- Have a friend hold the other end of the band and pull you in odd directions while you practice torso stabilization. This simulates walking a dog, or carrying packages and a squirming baby while trying to get in the door.

- Swing a hula-hoop around your waist. Try it again, swinging it around your arms. Try swinging the hula hoop around one arm while moving against the resistance of the band held in the other hand.

Not using abdominal muscles to control positioning during arm tasks is a common contributor to shoulder pain. By not using torso muscles to power the move, you may overload and over-rotate your shoulder. Over-rotation can occur in sports like swinging a tennis racquet, or in a high brace in kayaking, and in daily life. Reaching over the car seat for heavy items in the back seat without using supporting musculature frequently adds to rotator cuff injury. Use neutral spine and power the move with the abdominal muscles, not by levering the weight with the shoulder joint

Add balance and stability: Add balancing on one foot
Do any of the Ab Revolution bands and cable drills while standing on one foot. One foot training adds balance, strength, and stabilization training for core, legs, ankles, and feet.

Ab Revolution Bands and Cables for Training Throwing and Other Overhead Arm Activities for Sports

These drills practice using oblique (side) abdominal muscles to hold neutral spine for more speed and power during swinging and throwing.

If you allow the bad habit of increasing lower back arch, the fulcrum of the swing or throw becomes the shoulder and lower back joints (facets) instead of core and hip muscles. Shoulder injury and lower back pain can accumulate. Using neutral spine shifts effort off the joints and onto abdominal muscles for stronger and healthier exercise.

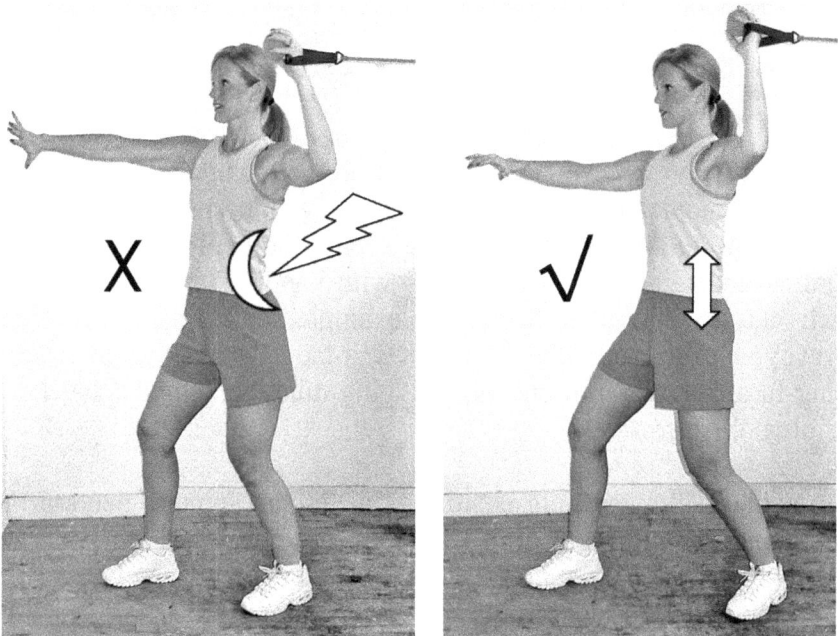

Left: Hyperlordosis, back arched, abdominals not in use. Right: Core in use to change lower spine posture to neutral, and power the throw.

1. Use cable pulleys or secure a stretchy band or tubing at about shoulder height. Face away from the resistance. Move further to increase resistance to desired amount.

2. Don't allow the resistance to pull your upper body backward into hyperlordosis. Don't tip the pelvis forward to assist the move. Maintain neutral.

3. Simulate throwing a ball or other object. Using neutral spine position, push off your feet, turn your hip, and swing the arm forward in a pitching and throwing action. Feel the pivot coming from your abdominal muscles not your shoulder or lower spine.

4. More range can come from the hip and upper spine extending, using abdominal muscles to hold lower spine neutral and power the throw.

Swinging A Medicine Ball, Kettlebell, India Club, And Other Heavy Objects

Swinging heavy objects has long been done in many cultures. Objects may be a medicine ball on a rope, bowling pin shaped clubs (India clubs) that are thrown, juggled, and swung, bolos (to sling stones for hunting and target practice), stones with handles (many names from each culture that uses them, for example, chikairashi, kettlebells, yirevoy, chishi, and others), the Kwan-tao (General Kwan's heavy kung-fu ax), heavy poi chains, swinging dumbbells, and other heavy training objects.

Use abdominal muscles to position your lumbar spine to neutral, then initiate action with your arm. Check if you increase lower back arch when swinging overhead, especially as the object swings behind you. Use abdominal muscles strongly to keep neutral spine.

Add balance and stability: Swing and throw while balancing on one foot

Do any of the Ab Revolution throwing and swinging drills while standing on one foot. Practicing on one foot adds balance, strength, and stabilization training for core, hip, legs, ankles, and feet.

Knife and Other Target Throwing

Use neutral spine and pivot the throw with more abdominal muscle flexion to increase speed and power, rather than arching the lower spine.

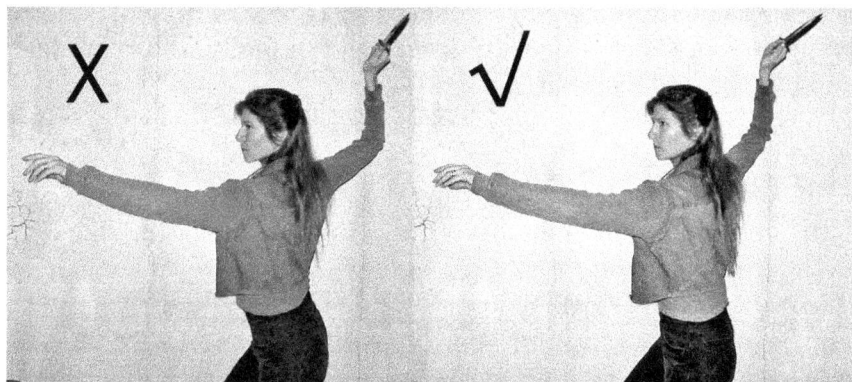

Left: Hyperlordosis. Pivot points shift to shoulder and spine joints. Right: Neutral spine makes a faster, more powerful throw. Abdominal muscles power the throw.

Done correctly, you should feel the effort shift to your abdominal muscles, and off your spine and shoulder capsule.

If you aren't sure how to move your spine to neutral, use the Part I section, "A Few Ways to Fix Hyperlordosis and Learn Neutral Spine."

Ab Revolution Neutral Spine For Archery and Other Target Sports

Recreational Archery

If you increase lumbar arch when drawing a bow, your chest and abdomen may protrude outward into the line of the bowstring. The bowstring can painfully hit your breast or body upon release. Straighten your stance to neutral spine to keep the front of your body out of the line of the bowstring.

Firearms Practice

One of several techniques in firearms shooting is to "lock out" a stance to the end range of the joints to steady the stance, including hyperlordotic lean-back of the upper body. Spine joints receive the impact of the firing. Locking arms straight is needed to prevent recoil from flinging the weapon, or your arms or hands, backwards to your face. However, it is healthier for the spine to hold steady firing using a solid neutral spine, rather than locked out while leaning backwards at end range of the spine. You should still be able to hold a steady shot, and you will shift the recoil from your spine to your abdominal muscles. If you are not strong enough for your device size, then strengthen yourself, but do not jeopardize safety of anyone.

If you are not sure how to move your spine out of hyperlordosis, use the Part I section, "A Few Ways to Fix Hyperlordosis and Learn Neutral Spine."

Ab Revolution Using an Exercise Ball

An exercise ball is an inflated or solid ball of various sizes that you can use to exercise and stretch in many ways. It is sold under any number of trade names. Because a ball rolls, exaggerated marketing claims are made of increased balance, muscle use, or posture during exercise. However, you can exercise or lie on a ball with little muscle use and with poor spine positioning.

Expensive desk chairs are marketed with the ball as the sitting surface, with claims that the ball makes you sit better or use more muscles. However, you can sit on a ball with as poor posture and as little effort as on most other surfaces.

Sitting on whatever surface is not a healthy pastime. It spends time in bent-forward posture. After a day of sitting at a desk, going to sit on weight machines, sit in yoga, or sit on a ball to lift weights does not change or reverse the many problems of sitting.

Crunches on a ball have all the same problems of postural impairment and lack of application to real life as crunches off the ball. Sitting on a ball to lift weights, and lying on a ball to do crunches on a ball are two of the least effective uses of a ball.

Used without understanding, the ball is just another gadget that does little, and reinforces the same poor habits as other exercises. The ball can be put to better use with functional exercises that strengthen and train your abdominal and other muscles to work the way you need for healthy positioning for sports and daily life.

All the exercises that follow work abdominal and back muscles at the same time, strengthen arms and legs too, and train healthy spine positioning. Try the following with safety and good judgment:

Neutral spine planks and pushups with both feet on the ball

- Hold a pushup position (plank) with hands on the floor and the ball at your ankles or under your feet. Tuck your hip to straighten spine position to neutral. Do not let your spine sag under your weight.

- As you progress, do pushups with feet on the ball and spine held straight. Going a little past neutral to straight gives more abdominal exercise. Keep your head in line with your back, not hanging down.

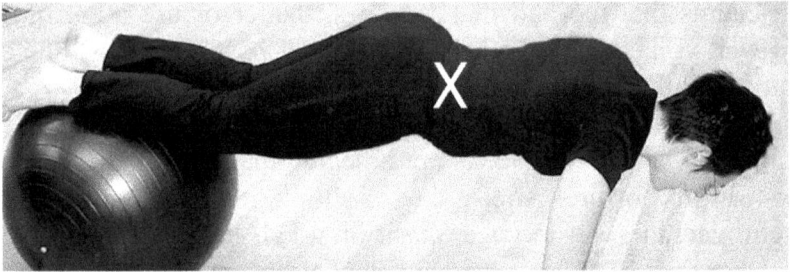

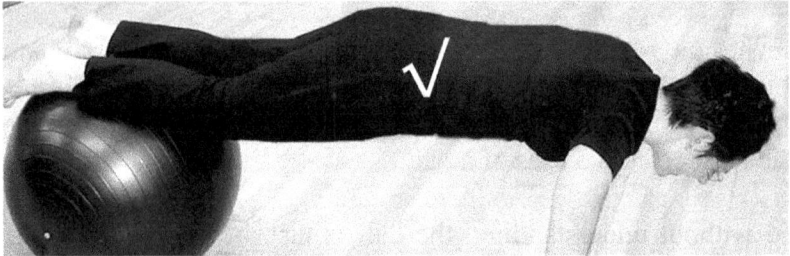

Top: Hyperlordosis. Anterior hip tilt, body weight sags on spine, shortened lumbar muscle length. Bottom: Straightened spine works abdominal muscles and practice avoiding hyperlordosis.

Neutral spine planks and pushups with one foot lifted

- In the pushup position with both feet on the ball and hands on the floor, lift one leg up and off the ball. Keep neutral spine. Hold as long as you can. Switch legs and hold.

- While holding the pushup position with one foot lifted off the ball, do pushups. Keep the hip tucked to straighten spinal position. Switch legs and repeat.

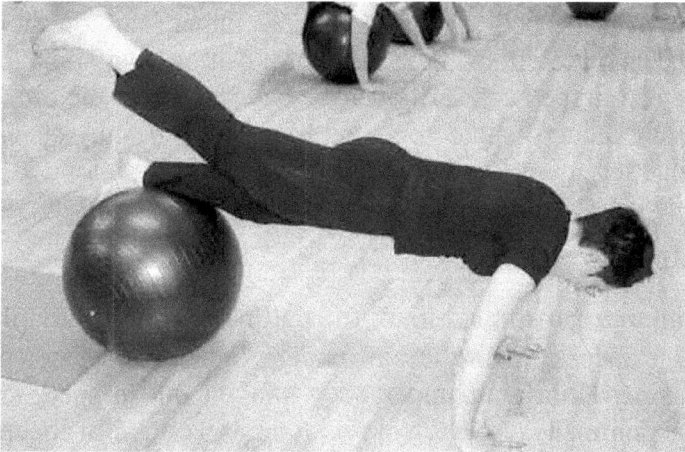

Lift one leg with straight spine positioning. Holding straight shifts body weight off the lower spine and onto the abdominal muscles. Try pushups this way.

Planks and pushups with one foot on the ball, one leg out to side

- Hold a neutral spine pushup position with both feet on the ball and both hands on the floor. Bring one leg off the ball 90 degrees to the side with toes and knee facing forward, and leg straight and parallel to the floor. This is the same "Peeing Dog" position as in the plank and pushup section, but with one leg up on a ball.

- To advance, repeat with the other arm lifted, holding all body segments straight and flat.

Side neutral spine with feet on the ball and hands on floor
- With both feet on the ball and both hands on the floor, turn your body to one side to stand sideways on one arm. Lift other arm up straight in the air. Hold straight body position as long as you can, then switch sides, keeping both feet or ankles on the ball.

Face up neutral spine, shoulders on a ball with feet on floor
- Lie on the ball face-up with your upper back on the ball and heels on the floor. Legs straight. Position your spine to neutral. Don't drape backward over the ball or bend at the hip. Hold the same neutral spine you need to train for healthy standing. Lift one leg up in line with your body and hold as long as you can. Switch legs and hold.

Face up neutral spine, hip on the ball with upper body plank
- Lie face up with the ball under your backside, not the lower spine. Hold your upper body straight out in space with your abdominal muscles. Hold as long as you can. Lift up one leg and hold as long as you can. Switch legs. Are you advanced? Lift both legs at once, lying flat and horizontal.

Side neutral spine, hip on a ball and upper body held in space
- Without using your arms, turn from the above position on the ball to lie on your side with the ball under your hip. Keep the side of your feet on the floor and your upper body straight out in space. Hold straight position as long as you can. For more, lift both arms over your head, biceps by ears. Advanced? Hold a weight in your hands. Roll to the other side without using your arms and repeat. Practice straight positioning.

Planks and pushups with hands on the ball and feet on the floor
- Put both hands on the ball and feet on the floor to hold a plank for increasing amounts of time. It is common to sway the

lumbar spine to make the plank easier. Hold neutral spine throughout.

- To progress, do pushups with hands on the ball, holding spine straight without letting it sway downwards. When you push upward, don't raise the upper body first, which increases lumbar arch. Lift the entire body straight upward as a unit.

- As you advance, roll to one side and balance on one arm at a time.

- Advance further by doing increasing dips on one arm until you can do side pushups on one arm.

Have fun using Ab Revolution for many moves on the ball.

If you aren't sure how to move your spine to neutral, use the Part I section, "A Few Ways to Fix Hyperlordosis and Learn Neutral Spine."

Using Ab Revolution To Fix Abdominal Twists

The use of twisting side-to-side holding a heavy bar or other weight is for torso muscles work to accelerate and decelerate the weight. If you use this exercise, check if you do it in a way that uses abdominal and back muscles to decelerate the weight before maximum twist, to prevent injury.

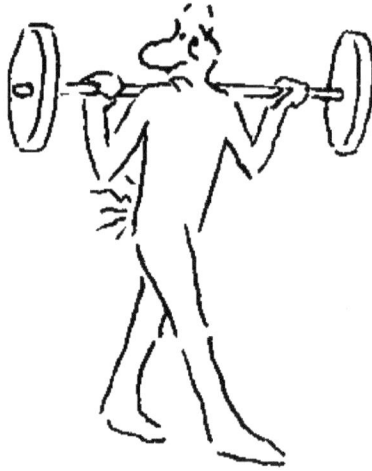

Beside a bent forward neck posture from a bar across the back of the shoulder (overcome by holding the weight in front), one problem comes from stopping the momentum at the end of each rotation with the vertebral joints, not abdominal muscles. Resulting rotational force (torque) on the spine can eventually strain, fray, and sheer discs and soft tissue, and overstretch tendons that hold muscles on bones and ligaments that hold bones together.

Instead of letting the rotation swing your body to the end range of your spine, decelerate using abdominal and torso muscles. Activities that require body knowledge of how to decelerate a swinging pivot include swinging a bat or racquet, swinging limbs in martial arts, some dancing, and rodeo activities, among others.

If all you want is pivoting exercise for side abdominals, one of many options is to use cable pulleys or a stretchy tube or band. No momentum continues the motion past the point to where you pull the band. Use movements that simulate and practice real daily life activities to make it functional exercise. Practice throws, punches, serves, paddling motions, swings, and anything else you need to train for better real life motion.

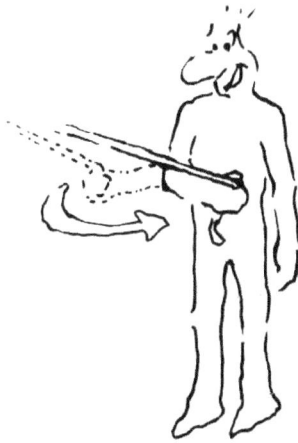

The "ab study" mentioned in Part III rated stretchy tubing low on abdominal muscle activation. One reason is that they used tubing while bending forward, rather than real life movements. Also, most people do not use much resistance on their band. To get useful, effective exercise, use a thick band, step away to increase tension, hold neutral spine against the resistance, use a wide range of motion, and go for the fun of the work.

A pivot-resisting exercise that is fun to do with kids or a friend is to stand with arms crossed over your chest. The second person grasps your arms or elbows, like holding a steering wheel or handlebars, and tries to "drive" and turn the wheel right and left while you resist. Both of you keep the body upright. Notice and fix if either partner hunches the shoulders, tenses the neck, or strains breathing. Practice relaxed breathing at the same times as strong movement, and then transfer that practice to daily life. To try this drill solo, hold a doorway, sturdy pole or pipe, or other hard-to-move object.

Ab Revolution for Punching

Hyperlordosis allows injurious force on the lower spine, not only when punching, but receiving a blow. Hyperlordosis also reduces punching force, because core muscles are not driving the punching arm. The fulcrum of the punch becomes the lower back instead of the muscles of the abdomen, chest, and hip.

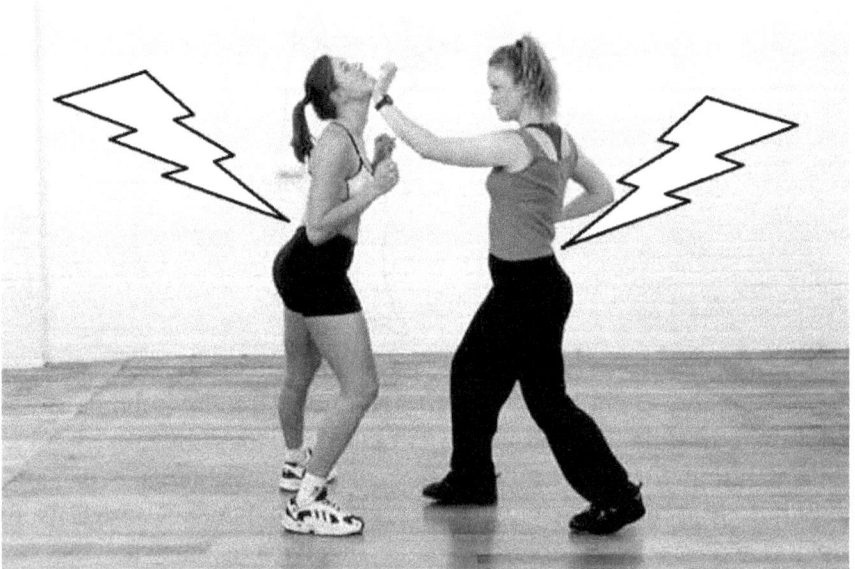

Punching in hyperlordosis increases compressive injury force to the lower spine and soft tissues in both puncher and receiver, and decreases force of the punch.

Training abdominal muscles for punching

1. Stand near a wall or other structure. Push against the wall with your fist with your arm extended.

2. To feel lower spine compression with hyperlordosis, allow the push of your arm to increase the inward arch of your lower back. Lean your upper body backward and tilt the hip forward in front. As you push increasingly hard, you may feel pressure or a familiar ache in your lower back. Don't do this if you already have back pain from overarching.

3. To correct spine position, tuck the hip under as if beginning a crunch without bringing your neck forward. Your pelvis and hip moves from tilted to vertical, from the top of the leg bone to the middle of the crest of the hip. You should feel lower back pain disappear, the effort shift to the abdominal muscles, and a new strength in your punching arm.

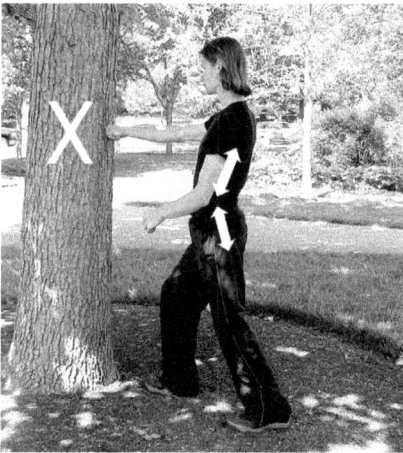

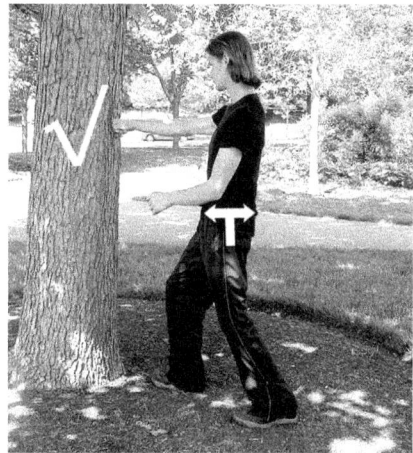

Left: Hyperlordosis. Hip tilted forward increases lower spine angle (arch) and injurious pressure, and reduces lumbar muscle length. Power of the punch lessens. Right: Neutral spine. Hip tucked from tilted to vertical. Upper body upright.

Initiate punching from the lower body, not the arm or shoulder. First, bring spine to neutral is if is not already. Bring pelvis and upper body vertical. Push off your feet, swing from the legs and hips, exhale, and feel the effort of your abdominal muscles as you extend your arm forward. Don't increase arch in your lower back at any point during the punch. Don't hunch or round forward. Rounding puts your chin closer for your opponent to hit.

Whenever you punch, use neutral spine. Hyperlordosis shifts effort from abdominal muscles to lumbar spine, and reduces punching power. When you change spine position from hyperlordosis to neutral spine while throwing a punch, you will feel lumbar pressure stop, and punching power increase immediately.

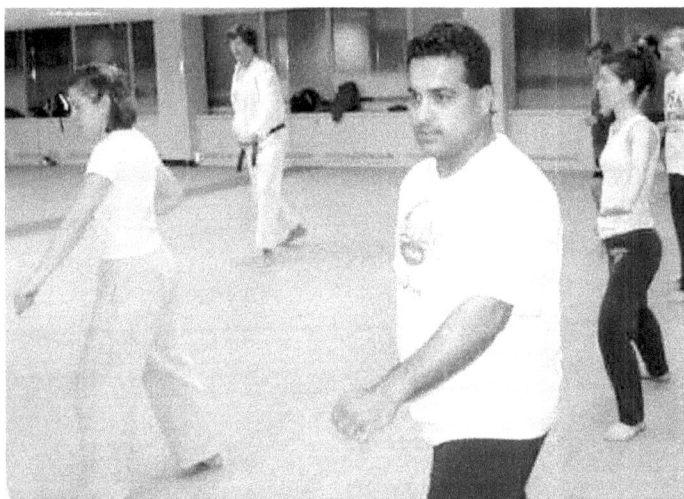

Can you spot the students not using abdominal muscles to control spine position in the karate class above? They are, first on the left, and on right to a higher degree.

Ab Revolution Punching Using Bands Or Cables

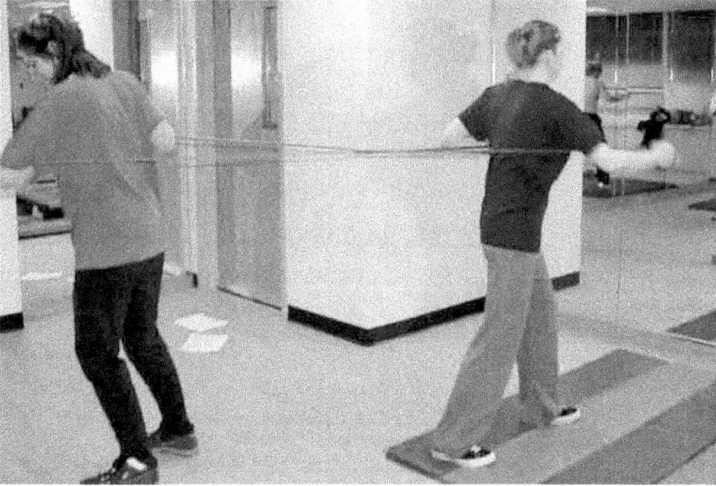

Both subjects in photograph above are leaning forward instead of standing upright. Leaning makes the exercise easier, in other words, less exercise. Stand upright as much as you can against the pull of all but the heaviest of bands, using neutral spine for increased abdominal work, and built-in postural training.

Leaning doesn't hurt the spine, but it does decrease core use for general weight training. Train to stand straight against resistance by using abdominal muscles.

1. Use a stretchy band or cable pulleys, secured around anything solid at shoulder height or above.

2. Turn your back to the resistance. Hold the band or cable under the arms, pictured above, if you need to prevent them from rubbing your skin.

3. Move further away to increase effort as needed.

4. Feel how to straighten your entire torso and hold neutral spine using your abdominal muscles. Maintain neutral spine position, not pulled backward or leaning forward.

Contract your abs first before pushing with your arm. Push off your feet and legs, turn your hip into the punch, then using your abdomen as the fulcrum lever your arm forward into a powerful punch. Breathe out as you punch.

Done correctly, you should feel any back pain disappear and the effort shift to your abs. You will feel your abdominal muscles working, but not tightening, to hold you straight against the load.

Save leaning against the load for extreme efforts and emergencies when you need the gravity assist. Otherwise, get the assist from your own muscles.

If you aren't sure how to move to neutral, use the Part I section, "A Few Ways to Fix Hyperlordosis and Learn Neutral Spine."

Using Abdominal Muscles For Pushing

All the abdominal muscles come into use for pushing things (anterior, oblique, and transversus) against heavy resistance. The following pushing exercise trains healthy, strong torso and back posture during pushing and slow powerful moves.

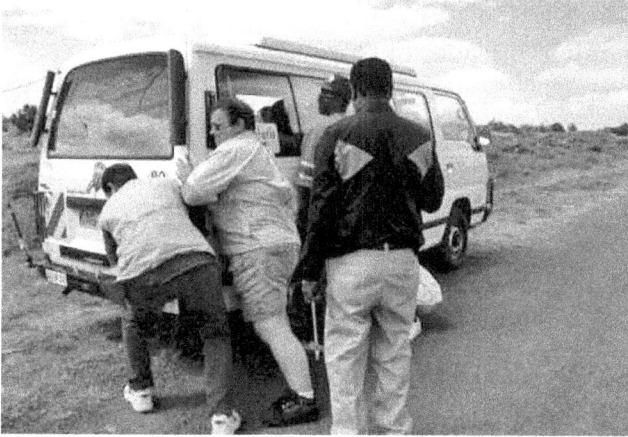

Prevent lumbar sway when pushing heavy objects. You will prevent lower back pain, and generate greater pushing force.

1. Stand with both hands against a wall. Begin pushing the wall with your hands, without bending your elbows. If you allow the push to arch your back, you may feel pressure, or a familiar ache in your lower back. (Don't do this if you already have back pain.)

2. Fix spine position to neutral, tucking your spine as if beginning a crunch but not bending your neck or upper body. You should feel back pain disappear, and a new strength.

3. Press off your feet, use your hips and abdomen as the fulcrum, and breathe out as you lever your upper body forward in powerful pushing action.

Ab Revolution for Kicking

In exercise, dance, martial arts, and other times when you lift legs for kicks and leaps, check spine position when kicking to the side and back. If you allow hyperlordosis, the fulcrum of the kick becomes the lower back joints instead of the muscles of the abdomen and hip. For the following, it is useful to be able to see yourself in a mirror.

Train abdominal muscles for kicking

1. Stand sideways to a wall at a distance to swing a side kick. Put the bottom of your foot against the wall, as if you just finished a side kick.

2. Notice if you let your back increase in arch. Begin pushing the wall with your foot without allowing your knee to give way. You may feel pressure; maybe the familiar ache in your lower back that you get from days (years) of bad posture habits. (Don't do this with increased arch if you have back pain.)

3. Fix your spine position by using your abdominal muscles as if beginning a crunch, but not bending your upper body forward. Reduce lumbar arch to neutral. You should feel back pain disappear and a new strength in your kicking leg. Do not curl the hip under, which increases pressure on the lower back discs, another kind of injury.

4. Practice your new neutral spine side kick. Don't allow your back to increase arch at any point in your kick. Don't hunch or round your back. Rounding is bad for your back and puts your chin closer to your opponent to hit.

Try the same technique for a back kick. Stand facing away from a wall. Put the bottom of your foot against the wall. Feel the difference between letting your back arch, and tucking enough to straighten your back without rounding it.

Ab Revolution Using Bands to Train Kicking

Train abdominal muscles for front kicking using bands

The following can be done by securing a cable pulley to your foot, or by securing a resistance band around your foot and the other end to something behind, or standing back to back with a partner with a long resistance band tied to one of each of your feet

1. Secure the band or cable handle around one ankle or foot as desired, making sure you are safely secured and standing with balance. Turn your back to the resistance of the band.

2. Step away to put tension on the band. Feel how to keep neutral spine against the backward pull on your leg. Stand up straight.

3. Make sure you keep neutral spine. Kick forward. Keep your standing heel down when you kick. Don't round your back forward to throw the kick. Hold straight.

Train abdominal muscles for side and back kicking using bands

*   Secure one end of the band or tubing handle around one leg. Turn to the side against the resistance of the band. Do side kicks while maintaining neutral spine.

*   Try the same technique for a back kick. Secure one end of the resistance to your foot. Stand facing wherever you have secured the other end. Move back until you get desired resistance. Kick backward. Feel the difference between letting your back increase in arch when you kick backward, and tucking enough to maintain neutral spine without rounding forward.

Using Abs for Supported Back Extension Without Compressive Hyperlordosis

There are activities in which you need to lean and extend backward, but still not let your spine compress with hyperlordosis, for example, for ballroom dancing, to take photographs from certain angles, for doing the limbo dance, and to reach awkward overhead repairs, among others.

What are flexion and extension?
Extension means increasing a joint angle. Elbow and knee extension makes a limb increasingly straight. Flexion usually is defined as making a joint angle smaller, such as bending elbow or knee so your hand (or foot) comes closer to your body.

Spine joints move in all directions. For most definitions, spine flexion is toward the front of your body, and extension is toward the back. Anatomically, full spine extension is considered holding the body straight (and fully extended elbow and knee joint are straight). Hyperextension means bending backward. For movement, "spine extension" means movement toward the back (rear direction).

Done right, hyperextension past the midline, does not compress, sheer, or fold the spine backwards under body weight. It can be a good feeling stretch involving a backward bending along each vertebra, and a good abdominal exercise without pain or high degree of sustained compression.

Difference between healthful extension and unhealthful compression of hyperlordosis
Healthy spine extension is different from compressive deformation of hyperlordosis in two main ways:

1. Good extension distributes stretch along all the vertebrae. It does not allow one hypermobile lower spine joint to fold backward while the rest of the spine does not participate in the range of movement.

2. Supported extension uses much muscular control to hold spine position to prevent compressive spine angles. The abdominal are used strongly to prevent body weight from folding the lower spine backward.

Check during your stretches and yoga poses that extend the back. Make sure you do not fold rearward at one lower segment, with the rest of the spine either unextended or still rounded forward (flexed). Good extension allows more stretch without compression of the posterior spine.

Extreme, compressed ranges are for occasional fun activities, or emergencies like carrying heavy people out of a fire at awkward angles. When used all the time for exercise, stretch, or daily posture, the compressed hyperextension of hyperlordosis eventually damages. Brain health comes from being aware of why you are using extension, how much, how often, and if in healthy or unhealthy way.

Supported Extension With Roman Chair Exercise
Roman Chair exercise, done without using abdominal muscles to prevent overarching, can compress and pinch the spine. To support the extension, strongly use abdominal muscles to decelerate as you extend backward. Don't hang your weight on your lower spine at end-range, but keep some uplift effort on the abdominal musculature.

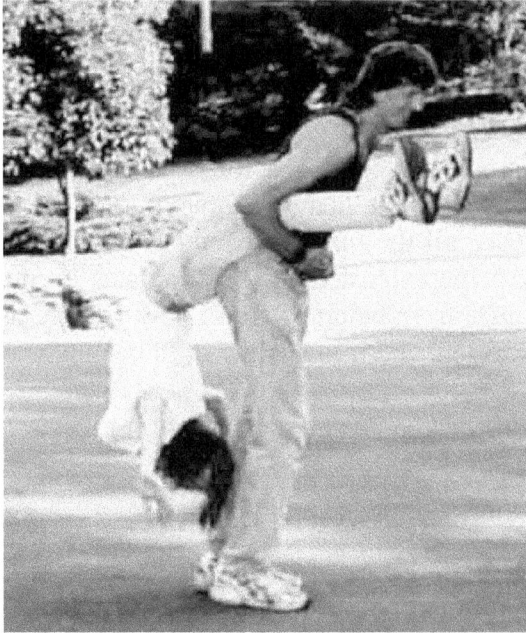

To advance, hold horizontal position with body straight for brief periods. Bad mechanics carries high risk of disc sheer and other damage. Be sure and supervised with more education that this brief paragraph.

Supported Extension For Headstands and Handstands
Use ab-supported extension for headstands and handstands to get range from extending the spine without compressing it.

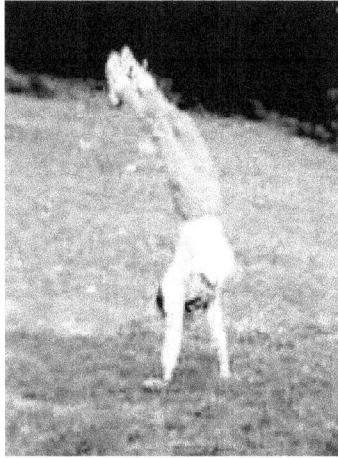

Spine is extended but not compressed, with technique to hold weight on the abdominals.

- Don't allow the weight of your legs to fold your lumbar spine backward at one segment.

- Use abdominal muscles to pull forward against the weight of the legs, preventing their weight from resting downward on the spine back, increasing joint and soft tissue compression.

- Get the extension range along the entire spine, rather than one easily mobile segment.

Extending makes balance easier, and is often used by beginners learning handstands. It is also used for various art forms where greater extension is sought for the look or the greater range of motion. Straight spine and body position for handstands is more balance practice, and was covered earlier in this section.

Ab Revolution For Stretching The Spine

Lying Down Extension Stretches

During face-down extension stretches such as "cobra" and "upfacing dog" check if you bend backward from one spine and neck area that easily bends, ignoring other areas. The lower spine and neck are already good at bending backward. They usually do not need more hyperlordotic effort. However, the upper spine is often kept rounded forward in modern life. It needs a beneficial stretch the other way.

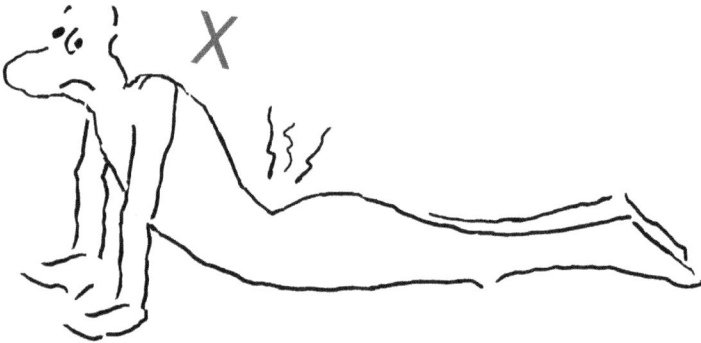

To fix this stretch:

- Use abdominal muscles to tuck the hip to neutral.

- Spread the stretch over the length of the spine, particularly the upper spine, letting it "unround." Only lift to where it feels like the stretch you want. Don't lift your chin. Keep neutral neck.

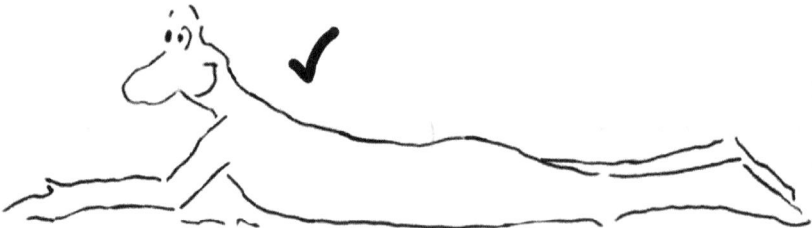

When you understand good extension, lift without using hands, getting extension and lift all along the upper back, not by bending backwards at the lower spine. Keep neck straight. The lift is from the upper spine, not the neck or lower spine.

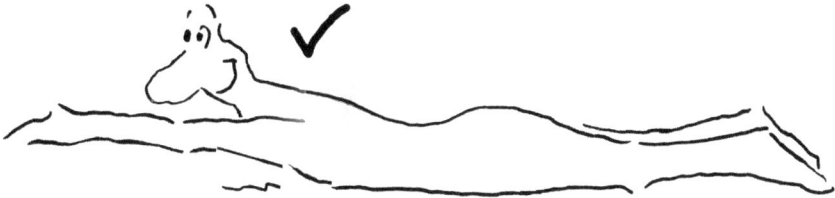

- Only lift the upper body to where it feels like the stretch you want. Don't force. Don't lift your chin. Keep neutral neck.

- The height you lift is not the benefit of the stretch. The idea is to get good extension and mobility from your entire spine without pinching or compressing any area.

- If you feel pinching in your lower back, tuck your hip. Move your upper body to a lower position until it feels comfortable and good.

If you are still uncomfortable, stop and see the section in Part I, "When Your Lower Back Hurts to Lie Flat Without A Pillow."

Prone lying with healthy extension unloads discs and can work for disc pain relief. Using the extension stretch in healthy ways can also be used to change a painful yoga routine to practice how to get healthy upper body extension during real life standing activities of looking and reaching upward.

Standing Extension Stretches

As with extension stretches lying down, the point is to get the range of motion from the upper spine.

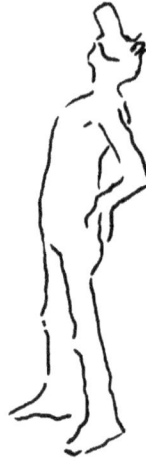

- Keep lower spine and pelvis neutral.

- Unround the entire upper spine (extend evenly), rather than folding backwards from the lower spine, or lifting the chin and folding backwards at the neck alone. It is healthier for the both the back and neck.

- Use abdominal muscles to pull forward enough to prevent the weight of your upper body from pressing downward on the lower spine.

Transfer the new healthier positioning to all your looking upward while standing.

More about supported spine extension is in the previous section, "Using Abs for Healthy Back Extension Without Hyperlordosis" including handstands, headstands, and roman chair exercises.

Using Ab Revolution For Balancing Stretches Like Yoga Tree Pose

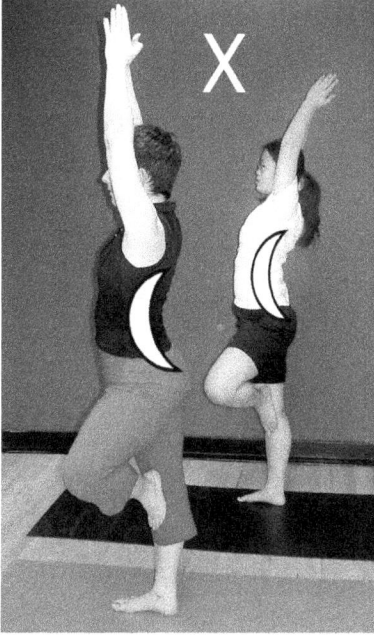

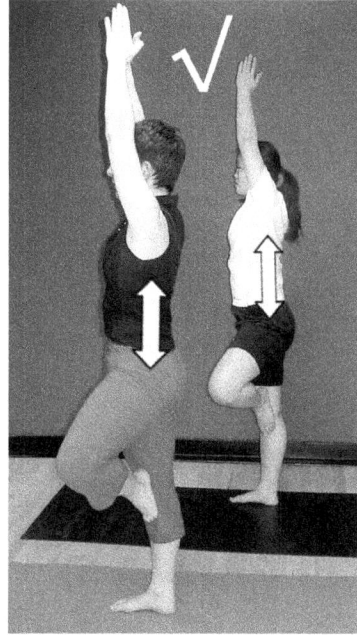

Left: Hyperlordosis. Lower back overly curved inward. Upper body leans backward (thoracic lean-back). Abs not in use.

Right: Same pose using abdominals to reduce hyperlordosis to neutral spine. Better stretch results in both hip and shoulder.

1. Keep neutral spine. Pelvis and upper body vertical.
2. Keep shoulders relaxed and down.
3. Instead of leaning back to raise arms, allow upper back to straighten for arm placement over ears.
4. Best placement for the raised foot is holding in the air, just next to the knee, not resting against it.

For advancement and fun, practice balance poses on a balance board, ball, roller, cushion, or other wobbly object for safe, higher training of neutral spine with balance challenge.

Ab Revolution For Stretching Arms Overhead

Be able to identify if you increase lumbar arch and lean the upper body backward when you stretch arms overhead. Hyperlordosis adds to lower back pain, and reduces stretch in the shoulder. Correct spine positioning to neutral spine and get more upper body range by "unrounding" the upper spine.

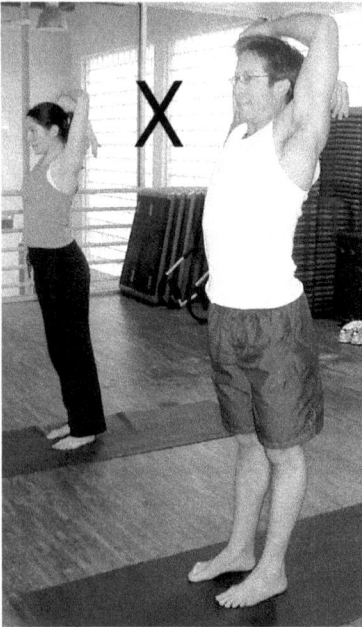

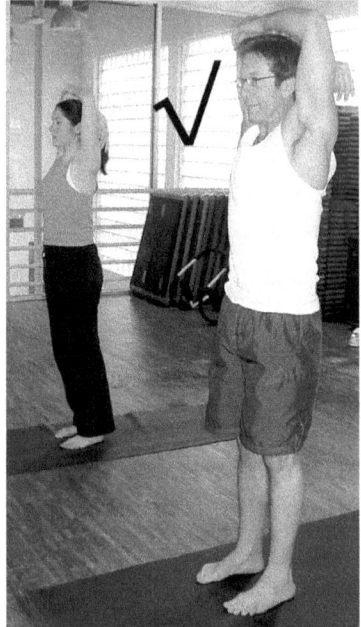

Left: Hyperlordosis. Less stretch on the shoulder, as range of motion comes from the lower spine arching and upper body leaning backwards, not from the shoulder and arm. Right: Same stretch using abdominal muscles to reduce hyperlordosis to neutral spine. Shoulder and arm stretch increases.

To learn better arm and shoulder stretch

1. Stand and lift arms high overhead and see if you allow your back to increase in arch. Notice if you lean the upper body backwards, lift the ribs, or tilt your pelvis.

2. With arms still overhead, flex your trunk as if starting a crunch motion to tuck the pelvis to vertical. Bring the upper body upright and vertical, not leaning backwards or curling your neck and head forward.

3. Feel the stretch move to your shoulder and triceps and pressure immediately leave the lower spine.

If you aren't sure how to move to neutral, use the section in Part I, "A Few Ways to Fix Hyperlordosis and Learn Neutral Spine."

Ab Revolution For Stretching Quadriceps and Anterior Hip

The front (anterior) hip and quadriceps stretch is a common stretch where you can lose the intended anterior lengthening, and add to lumbar compression pain by increasing lumbar curve.

Hyperlordosis is not caused by pulling the leg back, but allowing your hip to tilt forward and your spine to arch. The result is that the move comes from the lower spine shortening instead of the front of the hip and leg lengthening.

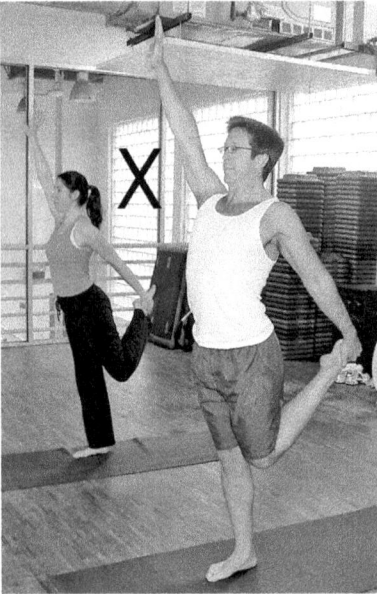

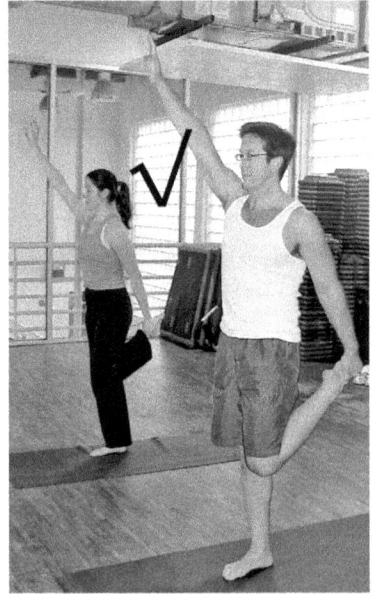

Left: Hyperlordosis. Anterior hip tilt and thoracic lean-back (tilting the hip forward and leaning the upper body backward). Stretch is reduced or lost on the hip and thigh. Right: Same stretch using abdominal muscles to straighten spine to neutral, and increase anterior hip and leg stretch.

To learn better quadriceps and anterior hip stretch

1. Stand on one leg and hold your other foot behind you.

2. Check if you allow your lower back to increase the inward curve. Notice if you lean the upper body backwards, lift the ribs, or tilt your pelvis.

3. Correct the area that needs correcting. For an anterior pelvic tilt, tuck the hip under, as if starting to do a lower body crunch. If the upper body is leaning backward, straighten to vertical. When you reduce lumbar curve, you will feel the stretch move to your thigh.

4. Don't pull your foot in toward your body. Extend your arm straight and push the foot away while you maintain lower spine position.

5. To be certain of the improvement, allow your lower spine to arch and feel the stretch lessen or disappear on the leg and anterior hip. Re-tuck and reduce lumbar curve to immediately feel better stretch.

6. As your flexibility improves by getting the range from the leg and hip muscles, not the spine, you will be able to bring the knee further behind the body.

By repositioning spine and pelvis, you should be able to make an immediate dramatic improvement in your stretch to quadriceps and the front of your hip.

Balance is important to health and independence. Practice balance safely using this stretch until you can stand on one leg.

If you aren't sure how to move to neutral, use the section in Part I, "A Few Ways to Fix Hyperlordosis and Learn Neutral Spine."

Real Athletes Need Neutral Spine

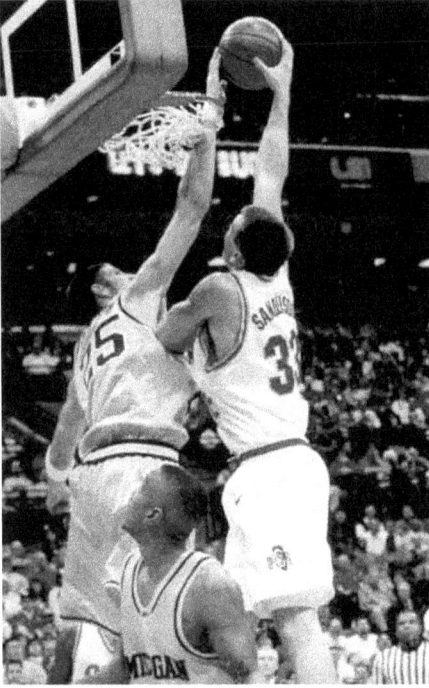

Both ball players in the photo at left show good use of abdominals to hold the spine in position while reaching upward to drive the dunk and power the block.

In the karate photo below, the black belts holding the board prevent lumbar sway using abdominals. The force of the punch is not levered onto their lower spine. The white belt has not learned this yet. Note how he incorrectly uses an arch to draw back the punching arm.

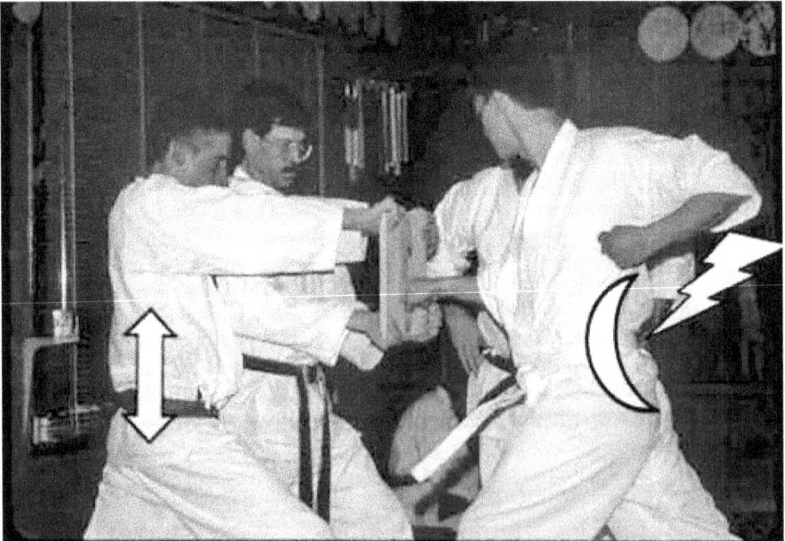

Part III
Understanding Abs
and
The Ab Revolution

What Exactly Do Abs Do?

More than other exercises, people seem to want to "do abs."
But why?

It is "something" to do with helping your back.
But what exactly do "abs" do for your back?

It's "something" to do with posture.
But exactly what?

It's something vague about "support."
What does "support" really mean?

What do abdominal muscles do?
A prevalent misconception is that using abdominal muscles means "sucking them in" "tightening them" or "pressing navel to spine." You cannot move or breathe in well that way. When you bend your arm, you don't tighten your muscles to do it. You can't tighten your legs and run well or comfortably. If you tighten your neck, it won't help your singing. Abdominal muscles move the body parts they attach to. Tightening abs does not make them do their job, does not change posture or let you breathe or exercise well.

Abdominal muscles connect your ribs to your hips along your front and sides. When you use your abdominal muscle, they pull your ribs and the front of your hip closer to each other, bending your spine forward, or to the front or side, depending which muscles you use more.

The real use of your abdominal muscles is when standing, to pull your ribs and the front of your hip closer to each other, to move your lower spine enough to come to neutral spine. When you stand and don't use your abdominal muscles, your ribs and hips move farther apart. Ribs lift up and/or the hip tips down. Either or both of these changes in body position exaggerate the normal inward curve of the lower back. Your lower back sways (overarches, becomes hyperlordotic).

Hyperlordosis drops the weight of your upper back onto your lower back, pressing down on your soft tissues and discs, and eventually irritating the joints called facets where each vertebra attaches to the next. Much facet pain and injury can result from the simple unhealthful positioning habit of hyperlordosis (too much inward curve in the lower spine).

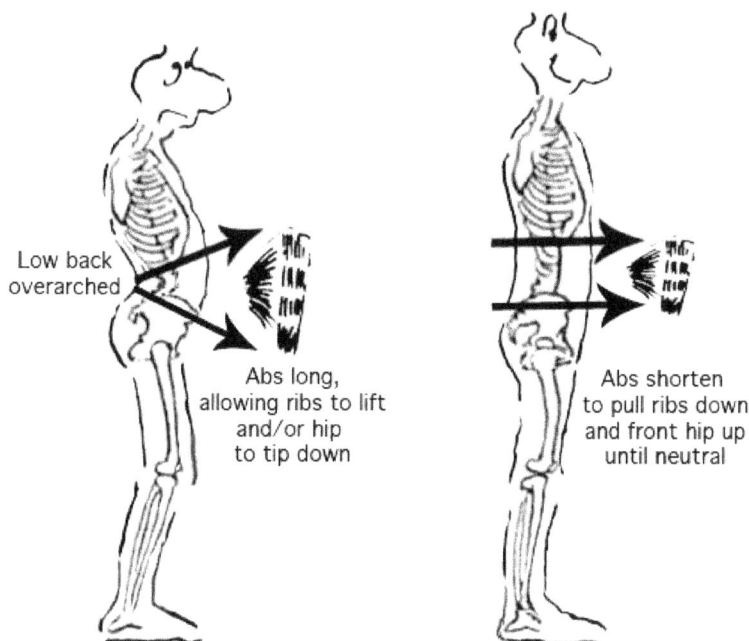

Left: Hyperlordosis. Thoracic lean (upper body leans backward, rib line tips upward) and anterior hip tilt (pelvis tilts forward and belt line tips downward). Both increase inward lumbar curve, which compresses and pinches the lower back.

Right: Neutral spine. Using abdominal muscles to pull ribs down to level, and tuck pelvis to neutral. A small inward curve remains in the lower back, not a painful exaggerated one.

What Do Gluteal Muscles Do?

A common statement is that you must squeeze or strengthen your gluteal muscles to fix spine posture. Those actions do not accomplish that, for several reasons.

Most obviously, squeezing muscles does not create movement, so cannot change any posture. Strengthening gluteal muscles will also not change posture from hyperlordosis to neutral. No strengthening causes you to move out of unhealthy posture automatically, and even if it could, the action of gluteal muscles is in the opposite direction. Gluteal muscles would cause the hip to push forward, which is one cause of hyperlordosis, not the correction for it. That also means that even if the gluteals were so weak that you could barely stand up, you still would not wobble or slouch into hyperlordosis from gluteal weakness.

Knowing muscle action will help you know why gluteal muscles don't work that way. Your gluteal muscles are several muscles of your backside. One function is to pull your upper leg backward, for example, when walking, to pull each leg behind you. The distance between the back of your hip and the back of your upper leg shortens. If you use gluteal muscles while standing (not tighten them in place, but use them to bring about movement) your pelvis will push forward. It will not change tilt as needed for hyperlordosis reduction, but push it forward. That is the opposite of what you want.

A common statement about a hip-forward posture is that it is due to weak gluteal muscles, and that strengthening the muscles would fix the bad posture. Various strengthening exercise are given, including lying on the back and squeezing the "cheeks" of the backside together as if squeezing a coin between them. Squeezing the gluteal muscles together is training a different movement direction than either pushing the hip and leg forward or back. It is also too little of an exercise to strengthen.

Another fallacy is that tight gluteal muscles pull the hip so that it pushes forward into bad posture. Gluteal muscles stretch to long lengths daily with sitting. If gluteals were so unable to stretch that they pushed the hip forward a few inches, they would be tighter than the short length needed for standing. In that case, they would be so tight that you could not sit down. You would tear your backside like splitting your pants. Tightness in the front of the hip can change hip angle to anterior tilt, but that is the opposite direction.

Strengthening muscles and bones and mind is good and helpful and fun and healthy, and so on. Strengthening gluteal muscles or any other muscles will not automatically make you stand in healthful position.

Don't squeeze abdominal or gluteal muscles. Squeezing or tightening any muscles hinders movement but doesn't create it. The motion of reducing hyperlordosis uses the abdominal muscles, not gluteals, to flex the lower spine until neutral.

Using Abs Doesn't Mean "Sucking Them In" or Making Them "Tight"

Using your abs does not mean "sucking them in" or "tightening them" or "pressing your navel to your spine."

Tightening and pressing are practically universal phrases to describe using abdominal muscles. They are incorrect and outdated. They are not the way to use your abs the way you need for real life movement.

Tightening is not how to use abs, or any muscles, for good posture. You can have poor posture, back pain, and an overly curved inward lumbar spine, even with "tight" abs (meaning clenching or holding extra muscle tension, not meaning lack of fat covering them).

To see why tightening is not how to use abs, try the following:
Bend your elbow to bring your hand up to your face. You didn't tighten anything.

Move your arm around. It didn't tighten (or shouldn't). You voluntarily move your arm to the position you want using muscles, not tightening them. Now move your torso side to side, then forward and back. You didn't tighten (or, should not tighten, it's unnecessary, unhealthy movement habits if you do). Moving your torso into good posture by using and core muscles is the same. It is voluntary movement to change the amount of bend and curve in your spine.

Now try tightening your abdomen, as commonly taught. Press your navel inward to your spine. Tighten the entire area. Now while holding tight and pressed hard inward, try to inhale to "belly breathe" as so-often taught as healthy normal breathing You can't, because abdominals are expiratory muscles. Tightening inhibits breathing. Moreover, walking around with "tight" muscles is a common factor in stress/strain-related muscle pain, and headache from habitually tightening upper body muscles. Tightening is not healthful or useful for daily activity

Next, stand in hyperlordosis / lumbar swayback, leaning the upper body backward or tilting the pelvis forward (don't do this if it hurts). Tighten or squeeze your muscles. Note that posture does not change.

Now stop tightening the area so that movement is unrestricted. Tuck your spine and hip to neutral and make upper body upright and vertical to reduce the hyperlordotic arch to neutral. See that "using your abs" is like any other muscle, to move your body.

Instead of lying on the floor and hunching forward to exercise your abs, train your abs to work the way you really need them—standing and doing all you do.

By using your abs to hold healthy spine positioning during all your activities, you will get free exercise and abdominal muscle training that benefits your life and helps your back. Simply strengthening abdominal muscles will not prevent this cause of back pain. Using the muscles to move into healthy neutral torso position is how it works.

This is new and different; a revolution in abdominal muscle and core use and training. It will teach you new thinking about abdominal muscles, and fun new skills to be fitter, healthier, and free from pain from hyperlordosis.

Why Do People With Hyperlordotic Back Pain Often Feel They Need To Bend Forward To Feel Better?

Constant forward bending isn't healthy for the spine. Why would someone feel better to bend over forward that way?

Many people hurt from excess inward lumbar curve that compresses and shortens lumbar structures. Bending forward briefly lengthens the crushed and shortened area. They feel better for that moment, because they stopped the reason they hurt (swayback) but only for that moment. When they return to standing in hyperlordosis, they shorten and compressg the lumbar area again until it hurts again. It is no mystery that pain returns.

The mistaken idea of "fixing" back pain with flexion (forward bending) exercises resulted in numerous unhealthful exercise and pain rehab programs which cause discs degeneration, hip pain, and hip dysfunction. Strengthening core or abdominal muscles does not fix the pain because it does not stop the cause. Stopping the painful bad posture, all the time, stops the pain all the time, and prevents it from coming back.

Other populations with narrowing of the spine, for example, some people with stenosis, also feel better to bend forward, as they open a bit of space in the rear of the vertebrae. They may keep bent-forward position all the time, creating new problems. They get pain when they increase lumbar curve trying to straighten up. For many of them, learning to make neutral spine possible through a little practice and specific stretching solves both problems.

See some solutions to get started with in Part I, "When Your Lower Back Hurts to Lie Flat Without A Pillow."

Is Hyperlordosis Natural?

People see slouching and hyperlordosis occurring often, and equate "common" with "natural."

Slouching your shoulders is common. It is a common cause of neck pain. It is natural? Wetting your pants is natural too, at first. Hitting people is natural for some. A little control, and life is healthier for all. Many people who believe hyperlordosis is natural also have pain and think it is "just the way they are made" without realizing it is a voluntary posture in their power to change.

Developmentally, which means during the ordered transitions from the completely straight spine of babyhood to childhood, spinal curves increase. During a brief period of childhood and sometimes into pre-adolescence, a lumbar curve overly increasing to hyperlordosis sometimes arises as a temporary developmental period, then transitions to the more stabile and neutral spine of teens and adulthood. Give children good examples and education so that they can grow to healthy adulthood through their many transitions. Teach them while young, so healthy information is ingrained. Trying to introduce and instill it later, it becomes "nagging."

For teens and adults, practice spine control until neutral spine becomes natural, and a usual, ordinary, built-in, customary, and normal movement stability habit.

Then it won't be natural to have back pain.

Ab Revolution Exercises Work Your Abs the Way You Need For Real Life - Functional Exercise

Many conventional ab and core exercises make you good at bending forward, moving in ways that have little to do with how you move or use those muscles in real life. For daily life, for most of what you do, abdominal muscles need to work nearly isometrically (at one length) to hold stable neutral spine, not to round your spine. You need to exercise your abs the way they normally need to work. This is called functional exercise. That means radically different exercises.

Ab Revolution exercises work your abs in functional ways, which means how you actually need to position your spine control when you stand, walk, run, carry packages, do exercise, sit, and go out and have fun.

Muscles can ache from fatigue at the end of a day. Most strengthening can quickly help to provide some margin to handle the demands of tiring life. However, not all strengthening is healthy over the long run. It is best to strengthen in healthy ways.

More important than how many repetitions you do, is understanding and using the concept of how abdominal muscles work to change spine and hip positioning. You need to use abs to adjust spine angles during exercise, and train your brain to transfer this body knowledge to all your daily activities. Doing repetitions and sets of conventional ab exercises without knowing and using neutral will not work your abs the way you need, and won't help your posture, your back, or your life.

Exercises don't fix causes of back pain. Use the repositioning taught in Part I to fix this kind of pain. Use Part II to increase ability, get stronger, get healthful exercise, have fun burning calories, for better physique, train functional abdominal use for healthy spine positioning, and practice back pain prevention.

Problems of Hyperlordosis During Exercise

- Swaybacked posture from tilting the pelvis forward (anterior pelvic tilt) interferes with normal walking and running mechanics. Your hips endure extra wear.

- Anterior pelvic tilt bends the hip forward (flexes and shortens) at the crease where the leg joins the hip. Anterior muscles are not lengthened to ranges needed for exercise and health. Increased lumbar angle shortens lumbar muscles length. Keeping muscles in shortened position tightens them, causing a cycle of tightness, poor posture, poor use, and pain.

- Hyperlordosis is sloppy technique and wasted effort. It does not effectively employ abdominal muscles. Why spend time exercising when you don't get intended results? You are missing a free workout of your core muscles and free built-in stretch for hip and back muscles.

- Hyperlordosis is a sign that you are not generating effective force in your limbs during arm or leg activity, because core muscles are not driving the limbs. See the sections on punching and kicking. Allowing the lower spine to slouch and increase inward curve under body weight is a weak, unfit posture, is injurious to the lower back, and is a marker of not using abdominal muscles.

- Hyperlordosis is often, unfortunately, thought of as normal, or relaxed, or cute. It is not healthy and not normal, even though common. Hyperlordotic, overly sagged inward lumbar curve, is seen in an astonishing number of fitness videos, magazines, books, and classes. The model may say "keep neutral spine," along with the usual (but incorrect) "tighten your abs." However, you may see that they sway their spine and tilt their pelvis in many exercises such lifting weights, holding a "plank," using the exercise ball, during leg lifts, and other exercises.

- Hyperlordosis is accepted as normal so often that it is mistaken for, even used to advertise, for fitness and trimness. However, it is a sign of unfit, unhealthy practices, tight hip, tight lumbar muscles, and/or not using abdominal muscles, and is a frequent and often missed contributor to lower back pain and tightness.

- Advertising uses hyperlordotic bad posture because sex sells. So does heroin. Notice when a display of slouching and lack of health is sold as fitness. Notice when you see "fitness" models standing or exercising with unhealthy overarched spine position. You may notice often, because this unfit posture is a common problem.

When Does Hyperlordosis Occur?

Check your lower back and hip position when you stand, walk, lift your arms, reach up, and look upward. See if you lean your upper body backward when you carry a load like a laundry basket, chair, or baby. Notice if you lean back to take photographs.

Many people cannot even straighten their shoulders to neutral from a rounded position, or drink a glass of water without leaning backward and increasing lumbar curve. Much lower back pain results, often thought of as a mystery, when it comes and goes; however it is from an easily changed bad posture.

Check if you allow hyperlordosis when standing in daily life. When exercising, check when doing pushups and planks, yoga poses, for squats and lifting weights. Increased lumbar curve makes the exercises easier because the abdominal muscles do not hold your weight. The weight is shifted to the spine joints called facets, and soft tissue, causing wear and aches. You miss the exercise and health benefits, don't work your abdominals, and are adding to back pain, even if you think you are exercising to stop it.

Reducing lower spine inward curve to relieve lumbar compression is the reason for the footrest in many pubs. After long standing at the bar, many people notice that their lower back aches. The reason is not long standing, but long standing in swayback. When people put one foot up on the footrest, they often unwittingly tuck the hip under along with it, reducing lumbar arch. Back pain reduces immediately. You can do this yourself without the bar, by reducing a too large inward curve to neutral. Abdominal muscles help your back by moving the spine out of painful position, not through crunches or strengthening.

What Is The Difference Between Lordosis, Hyperlordosis, and Swayback?

The word "lordosis" originally meant the normal slight inward curve of the lower back in neutral spine. Hyperlordosis means too much lordosis. Unfortunately, painful arch was often referred to as "lordosis" mostly for the location of the painful arch. That further became confused when texts referred to "painful lordosis" then practitioners started using the terms interchangeably. That is why you can read that lordosis is bad and that it is good, or that you need lordosis, which made some instructors think that meant you need more curve, and so on. Lordosis means small normal curve.

In this book, hyperlordosis means too much lordosis. More terms for this same slouching posture are swayback, lumbar overarch, and too much inward lumbar curve or sway.

Hyperlordosis is not a medical condition or a structural problem that needs drugs, treatments, surgery, or weeks of exercises to fix. It is a bad posture habit. It is quickly changeable and preventable.

What About Ab Rocking Devices?

Various rocker devices on the market are little cages in various shapes to rock you for crunches. They attract users because they make crunches easy, and crunches are familiar. Problems are that easier means less exercise, and that crunches aren't the best exercise for abdominal muscles or the rest of you.

Doing crunches with or without a device does not train you to use your abs the way that you need for daily life. It is not a functional exercise. The crunching motion of the devices promotes the same round-shouldered, round-backed, hunched-over poor posture as crunches. Even following instructions to keep the neck straight, the torso still curls. Most people already stand, walk, and exercise round-shouldered. The last thing they need is to exaggerate and practice that posture as a deliberate exercise.

Devices that are used to sit and curl forward against resistance have the same problems as crunches with the added problems of sitting, and sitting bending forward. Sitting has never been a healthy thing. It is a shame when people sit to exercise, and worse, pay to sit to exercise. Sitting bent forward is known as a higher load on the lower spine than even standing bent forward.

This book teaches ways to use your abs for good posture and effective use of abs during normal activity instead of crunches. Try The Ab Revolution exercises in this book instead. It is more effective not to do crunches, and instead, strengthens muscles in healthier ways and for the daily life positioning that relives back pain.

What About Ab Machines?

Abdominal exercises will not change your posture. Strengthening does not fix causes of most pain. If you are trying to fix back pain or posture, use Part I.

For people wanting abdominal exercise, machines are often used in ways that don't use the abdominal muscles. If you allow your spine to sag into hyperlordosis, your body weight hangs on the spine joints called facets, compressing the spine and soft tissues, eventually causing wear and pain, and reducing exercise on the abdominal muscles.

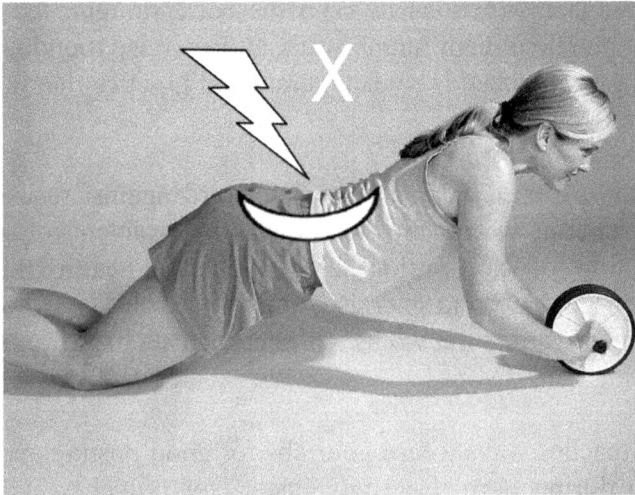

Hyperlordosis. Body weight hangs on the spine joints.
Abdominal muscles not in use.

To use any of the variety of ab machines so that you use your abdominal and core muscles, tuck your hip under until neutral spine or just past it. Straighten your torso. You will immediately feel your abdominal muscles work. Done properly, hyperlordotic pressure on the lower back will be relieved.

For more effective exercise, stay off your knees. Hold position on the hands and feet, not hands and knees.

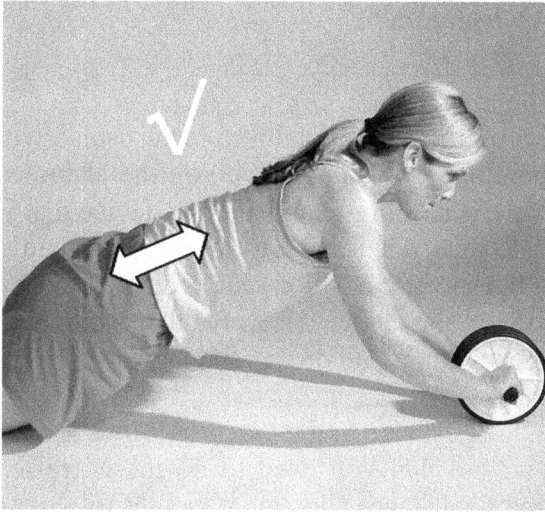

Go slightly past neutral to completely straight to feel abdominals in use, and pressure relieved on the spine. Instead of an expensive machine, you can use a simple wheel, or two roller skates, or a slippery floor with socks on your hands and feet. Stay off the knees for better training.

One way to remind yourself of how to do the hip tuck for using ab machines is to tuck while on hands and knees. Feel how your backside rotates downward and the spine lift upward until the inward curve lessens. Hyperlordosis correction is taught in Part I in the section of drills to learn neutral spine.

Practice to move your spine out of unhealthful sagging position without squeezing or tightening gluteal (or any) muscles. Keep your head in line with your body, not tilted downward or pinched back at the neck from lifting the chin instead of straightening the upper body.

Use a mirror to watch your posture in side view.

The point is to transfer practice and knowledge of how to change spine position to neutral spine to when you are standing.

What About Ab Isolators?

Several products on the market claim to better isolate your abdominal muscles and therefore (somehow) give you the abdomen pictured on the package. There is nothing in an isolating device that you cannot do without it. For instance, advertising for one device claims to hold your feet and legs in the specific position required for crunches. You can do that yourself without the device. However that would still produce the same hunched posture that you don't want anyway.

Some devices add resistance to the exercise. More resistance increases the muscle activation that you need to do the exercise, in the same way, carrying extra packages adds more weight for your arms to work against. There is nothing secret or scientific about doing more work to get more results. You can hold a weight or your body weight, taught in Part II retraining drills.

Most importantly, they do not work your abdominal muscles the way they work for upright daily life, or teach you that is even needed. In addition, isolating a muscle is not helpful to your real life. Life is a multi-segment activity. Plenty of people with muscular backs and abs from isolating them in gyms injure themselves opening windows. Plenty of people run miles on treadmills then sprain their ankle when walking on real earth. They are not used to using their body in a multi-functional, cooperative manner the way they need for real life. Similarly, people who do crunches in every workout and use every ab machine, often still stand in hyperlordosis, not using their abs, and putting undue wear on the lumbar spine.

What About Electronic Ab Zapper Belts?

"Watch TV while motorized stomach vibrator burns more calories than 500 sit-ups a day"

"Use electronic stimulating muscle contractor to get more muscle contractions than hundreds of sit ups"

Many advertisements for abdominal devices sound good, but are they true?

Early abdominal devices were little more than vibrators. They do not burn extra calories. Advertisers made claims comparing the relative number of calories you would burn in a longer time to a shorter one. In two hours of sitting in front of the television wearing the device, you would burn more calories than during the theoretical 15 to 30 minutes it would take to do the sit-ups, with or without a vibrator strapped to your abdomen. Burning calories is your normal metabolism at work to breathe, be alive, process body function, and do all you do. Claims of increased heart rate from electric stimulation do not necessarily mean any change in metabolism or more calories burned. There is far more to metabolism than heart rate.

Other devices stem from electrical muscle stimulators (EMS) used in physical therapy to passively contract muscles atrophied from paralysis or wasting diseases. These devises have been around for a long time. There is muscle contraction but not enough to produce the results claimed.

What About Miracle Liquids and Fat Burners?

Many products claim to burn fat while you sleep. Some claim to give a workout so intense that you burn fat for hours after you finish exercising. Other products are pills called "fat burners" but may not actually claim to burn any. It is marketing.

Everyone burns fat when they are asleep. When they are awake too. Metabolizing stored fat is part of your round-the-clock energy production for all body functions, whether you drink miracle potions or not. Advertising could just as honestly claim that if you stare at their special dot you will burn calories in your sleep. Don't pay money for that because you won't burn *extra* calories. You burn calories staring at a dot because you would burn calories anyway to breathe and live. You burn some fat 24 hours a day as part of being alive at all.

When you exercise, no matter what device you use, or potion you drink, you increase metabolism, which means total body energy use, to meet increased exercise needs. Metabolism returns to resting levels after you stop exercise, but takes time to return to resting levels. Any product can truthfully claim to coincide with increased calorie burning after a workout. Don't pay money for that because any run, bike, swim, or exercise will do the same.

Pills called "fat burners" are often stimulants and substances like them. They do not selectively find and eliminate fat cells. Increased heart rate from pills does not mean change in metabolism or more calories burned. There is more to metabolism than heart rate. Stimulant compounds can have harmful effects from nervousness and grouchiness to heart trouble and inability to exercise safely in the heat. Regular use makes you unable to function well without them.

Dancing, skating, playing, biking, and other fun ways to move will "pick you up" more effectively and safely than stimulants, will burn more calories, and keep you happier and healthier in the long run.

What About Neoprene Waist Bands?

Various products state that they "take off inches" just by wearing them. That have intriguing names like "waist support," "muscle support," "flab zapper," and "waist shrinker." However, the name of a product is not required to be what it actually does. They are only names. Vague and inflated claims may also be made.

Commercial garments are a neoprene or other tight elastic band to wear around your waist (or thighs, or hips, or wherever). The band squeezes you, temporarily shrinking your circumference through simple compression while wearing them and briefly afterwards.

The garments have nothing to do with toning or supporting the muscles, sweat loss, weight loss, or body fat loss. They compress, temporarily. You may notice that when you take off socks that are tight at the ankles, that there is a dent around your leg from the sock band. The elastic sock compressed your flesh leaving that area temporarily smaller. Your leg returns to normal circumference quickly. The same thing happens with neoprene waistbands. It is a not a true size change.

How Do You Flatten Your Abdomen?

Many people deliberately stand in swayback so that their abdomen curves outward in front. Exercises often done in gyms teach or encourage it. This is the opposite of the intended flatter abdomen. Use neutral spine, so that you do not curve the front of your body outward.

No exercise selectively removes fat from a specific part. That myth is called "spot reducing." No ab exercise removes fat from your abdomen, despite marketing claims. If spot reducing worked, people would have thin mouths from talking, speed skaters would have small legs, and the repeated act of chewing and swallowing lots of food would make your face thin.

Using up more calories to exercise than you eat, eventually burns stored body fat. To lose fat, including fat from your abdomen, go dance, run, swim, bike, row, skip, skate, jog, ski, run, walk, dig, play, and move in general. Do weight training to build muscle and burn calories from the exercise. Get out and have fun.

Conventional abdominal and core exercise alone won't teach or train you to stand properly to prevent your back from increasing inward curve and your abdomen from increasing outward curve. It is not "sucking in" or "tightening" that flattens an abdomen in healthful way. It is stopping hyperlordosis, by moving your torso into healthy neutral position that reduces the outward abdominal curve. After that, fat reduction is up to your healthy lifestyle.

How Do You Get "Washboard Abs?"

All the Ab Revolution exercises in Part II can show you how to work your abdominal muscles more than with conventional exercises. These drills also work the abdomen and back at the same time, giving your back and body healthy work and definition too.

The Ab Revolution teaches how to use muscles for real life. You learn to use muscle groups and body parts together, the way actually needed in real life, a bonus that works arms and legs, upper and lower body, while getting an abdominal muscle workout to help total physique.

You can use Ab Revolution exercises together to create a workout to burn calories as part of fat reduction in healthy ways that allows you to see the good results. Then there is less fat to hide your rippled abs.

Bands of fibrous tissue called fascia run at intervals across your abdominal muscles. Doing abdominal exercise will enlarge the muscles enough to extend a bit through the fascial bands giving a more "washboard" or "ripple" or "six-pack" effect. However, the visual appearance of abdominal muscles does not mean a person is healthy, has strong muscles, or uses the abdominal muscles to hold healthful spine positioning to move in healthy ways.

Use your muscles for real life outside of the gym—moving, balancing, lifting, reaching, jumping, throwing, dancing, and having fun. Consciously use your abdominal muscles hold your spine in neutral all the time without slouching into hyperlordosis.

Strong abdominal muscles may not be apparent if body fat covers them. Don't diet in unhealthy ways to get a cosmetic effect of abdominal muscles. Eat healthful meals. Cut out junk food. You will save money. Keep moving in fun, healthful ways. Dieting without exercise may reduce visible fat, but leave you without the important health benefits of exercise and movement.

How Many, How Often?

When to do Ab Revolution?
Use the neutral spine positioning in Part I all the time for standing, walking, running and going about your normal day. Exercises and retraining drills in Part II can be done any time, or everyday.

How many of each Part I exercise to do?
The idea is to learn neutral spine then use it. If that takes you a single try, then you have learned what you need.

How many of each Part II exercise to do?
Start with as many of each as you can in healthy position. Work up to more. The idea is to learn neutral spine right away then use it for as much exercise as you can do. Then continually increase abilities.

Many easier ones or fewer harder ones?
Regularly lifting weight that is so heavy that you can only lift it a few times builds mostly strength. Lifting lighter weight for a long time builds more endurance. You need both for daily activities, and getting through the day with healthy posture without a tired, achy back. For many people, their own body weight is so heavy relative to their ability that it provides enough resistance to build strength, for example pushups. As you strengthen, you'll be able to do more repetitions. Gradually add external weight, building both strength and endurance.

How fast or slow?
Working muscles slowly gets them good at slow movement. That is good for carrying things and pushing cars (if you also trained to be strong enough). It will not make you able to do fast movements needed for real life, like throwing, catching falling objects or children, swinging a bat or racquet, punching, blocking punches, or anything where you need your strength quickly. Practice exercises both quickly and slowly to maximize real life abilities. Practice how to be safe while moving at speed.

"Ab-Only" Exercises Are Not Functional

There are two main problems with doing conventional bending forward abdominal muscle exercise programs or "abs" classes with intention to reduce back pain or injury.

Abdominal muscles and back muscles are different muscles. Doing conventional abdominal muscle exercise does not work your back muscles, in the same way that walking does not make your arms strong. To strengthen your back, you have to work your back muscles with exercises that contract them in ways you need for real life, and in ways that do not add injury while strengthening. These kinds of functional exercises are in Part II. It is true that using abdominal muscles to reposition your spine out of an unhealthy arch stops lumbar pain from overarching, and there is a small effect on the back muscles called co-contraction. However, saying that forward bending abdominal exercise strengthens your back muscles is not true.

Doing conventional forward bending abdominal exercises adds to rounded shoulders, rounded upper back, upper crossed syndrome, and other upper and lower back pain. The chronic forward rounding puts unhealthy compression on discs, vertebrae, and nerves that exit the vertebrae. Forward slouching, from sitting rounded and exercising rounded, overstretches your back muscles and slowly pressures discs to bulge outward. Keeping your back muscles, or any muscles, lengthened by poor posture weakens them.

Habitual rounded forward poor posture is something people are usually already good at, and spend a large portion of the day doing. A common approach is to do conventional abdominal exercises by bending forward, then turn over to do a few back extension exercises. Doing back extensions will not undo a day of unhealthy forward bending. A better approach is to use Ab Revolution exercises in this book to exercise back and abdominal muscles at the same time, in functional ways, and to use healthy spine positioning for all you do.

What About "The Ab Study?"

A fitness industry survey compared 13 of the most common abdominal exercises and ranked them from most to least effective in producing abdominal muscle activity. It is a common assumption that weak abs are somehow connected to back pain, so it is often concluded that therefore strengthening the muscles is what is needed. This approach hasn't been working. There are several reasons why:

- An exercise may exercise a muscle, yet at the same time promote injurious posture and not be good for the rest of you. Smoking does "work" to lose weight but it is not a healthy way to do it, crunches and forward rounding abdominal exercises "work" the abs, but are not a healthful way to do it.

- Even if an exercise activates abdominal muscles, it still may not be useful for how you move in daily life. You don't hunch forward for daily activities. You do need your abs to help you to stand and walk upright without arching and sagging backward. Crunches and other exercises tested in the study don't train that. Posture and muscle use are not automatic. Strengthening a muscle does not train it for how you need it to work.

- Strengthening abdominal muscles will not automatically change spine positioning for healthy use in sports and recreation, or for back pain control. Plenty of muscular people have poor posture and much back pain.

The Ab Revolution teaches a different approach to abdominal muscle use, gives exercises that effectively develop your abs, and shows you how to transfer use of abdominal and other core muscles to daily life. Even if you don't care about posture or back pain and want only the cosmetic results of strong abs, use the Ab Revolution exercises in Part II for effective workouts.

What's Wrong with Crunches?

The most important use of abdominal muscles is when you are standing and going about your life. Crunches don't work your core muscles the way you need for real life. Crunches don't train your core to hold your spine in neutral position the way you need for pain free activity the rest of the day. They are not functional exercise, even when done "properly."

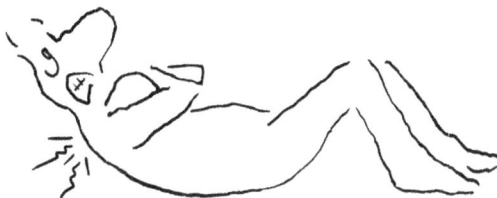

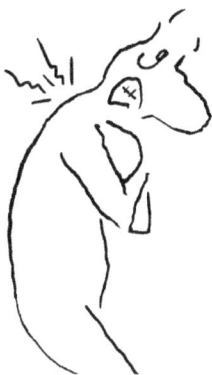

Look at crunches sideways and see how it would look to stand and live in that same position. Many people spend their life rounding the spine during most of their day sitting and working, then exercising that same way, until rounded position becomes accustomed, and increasingly difficult to straighten.

In real, daily life, your abdominal muscles need to work isometrically — at one length — to hold your torso upright, instead of allowing hyperlordosis. Crunches don't train you for that, no matter how strong the muscles become. Crunches make people, who likely spend much of their day already bent over a work area, practice that same position, which may be mechanically promoting the back and neck pain they think they are doing crunches to prevent.

Conventional abdominal exercise does not change hyperlordotic bad posture, or any posture. This is why most conventional abdominal exercises don't stop the cause of this kind of back pain. People do crunches all the time but don't know they are supposed to use their abdominal muscles in real life when standing to prevent the their lumbar spine from the injurious posture of hyperlordosis.

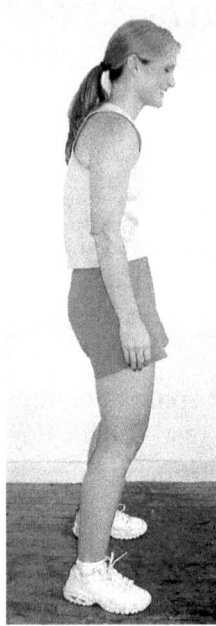

Crunches practice rounding forward. Most people do not need to practice such a position in real life. A small population who have conditions which cause the body to remain pulled and arched backwards stiffly, can benefit by practicing using abdominal muscles to pull and try to curl forward to gain needed spine flexibility and muscle use.

For most everyone else, instead of crunches and other abdominal exercises that use forward bending, in the belief it will relieve back pain, use abdominal muscles in the way that stops the hyperlordotic position that causes the pain — while standing, all the time, to reduce an overly large inward lumbar curve to neutral spine. You will train healthy spine position at the same time that you get free, built-in abdominal muscle training all day.

What Are All the Muscles Called?

Abdominal muscles are named for their layout in your body—where they connect to bones and to each other. Abdominal muscles don't work separately. They work in combinations. That is why it is good to work them together in functional exercises as described in this method.

Rectus abdominis

The muscle that runs vertically up the front of your abdomen is your rectus abdominis, which in Latin means "the straight abdominal." Your rectus abdominis starts on the front of your pelvic bone (lower front hipbone) and continues upward to attach to where your middle ribs (fifth, sixth, and seventh) come together in front. Not all the rectus fibers run up the muscle. There are three, sometimes four intersections across it. You can see these lines in trim people. Using your rectus abdominal muscle so that it shortens pulls your ribs and hips toward each other to bend you forward or prevent leaning backward. Preventing the upper body from leaning backward, and the pelvis from tilting, is how the rectus abdominis (and other abdominal muscles) prevent the hyperlordosis that creates back pain. The rectus muscle does not automatically create your posture or prevent pain by any tightening or by virtue of being strong, in itself. Pain prevention is direct, by using abdominal muscles to pull your ribs and pelvis toward each other enough to reduce a painful lumbar angle to healthful angle.

Obliquus externus

"Oblique" means slanted or not straight. Your oblique abdominal muscles run diagonally across your sides. If you put your fingertips at the top of your pants pockets, your hands line up in the direction of the outer set called external obliques. External oblique muscles begin as broad muscles on each side of your lower eight ribs. The outer external obliques on each side fuse together in a tough band in a nice line down your front under your front or rectus muscle. The deeper external oblique fibers run almost straight down to your hipbones.

Your obliques work together in fun ways. When the external oblique fibers on your right side contract, they pull your right side closer to the middle of your pelvic bone so you twist to the left. To control posture, you use your right obliques to resist forces that would twist you to the right. When you contract your left external oblique, you twist to the right (or prevent twisting to the left). When you contract both, you bend forward or prevent bending backward. An important function they have when contracting together is to keep your hip from tilting forward in front. Preventing tilting and arcing is how your external oblique muscles help prevent back pain. Pain prevention comes from using your oblique muscles to move to neutral spine, not from tightening or doing exercises.

Obliquus internus
Your internal obliques lie under your external obliques in the opposite direction. If you cross your arms over your abdomen, your fingers assume the direction of the internal fibers. Internal obliques begin at your hipbone and angle upward to your lower three or four ribs.

Your right internal oblique contracts to pull the middle of your ribs to your right hip, twisting you to the right. The left internal oblique twists you to the left. The right external and left internal oblique work together to twist you left. The left external and right internal work together to twist right. Contracting them all helps you bend forward, prevent arching backward, and prevent your hip from tilting forward in front. All the oblique muscles can resist forces that would make you want to slouch or twist in bad postures.

Transversus abdominis
Your innermost and thinnest abdominal muscle, the transversus, goes across your abdomen to help compress it for actions like breathing out fully, shouting, and childbirth. You can feel it when you breathe out as completely as you can. It is not the case that tightening the transversus like a girdle will prevent lower back injury when lifting or sitting.

Although a popular assumption that the transversus must be tightened, Dr. Stuart McGill, a major name in spine research, published that "drawing in" the abdominal muscles ("press the navel to spine") is detrimental to health of the lower back, and that tightening the abs impedes normal movement. In a paper in the *Archives of Physical Medicine Rehabilitation* (2007 Jan;88(1):54-62) he wrote, "There seems to be no mechanical rationale for using an abdominal hollow, or the transversus abdominis, to enhance stability. "

More importantly, tightening by itself will not position your spine in any way that prevents injury. It will not prevent you from slouching backward, or rounding forward, while lifting, both of which can accumulate injury to your back. Back pain protection comes from repositioning your spine by using, not tightening, your abdominal muscles to prevent slouching into unfavorable angles. Moreover, when you hold the transversus tightly, you increase your blood pressure, and cannot breathe in fully or properly (belly breathing) because the major purpose of this muscle is to produce exhalation.

The transverse abdominis is usually one of the muscles that people who do yoga (yogis) tighten and involve in doing "locks" along with the pelvic floor muscles. It is sometimes asked in yoga and other classes if the TrA (transverse abdominis) is one of the pelvic floor muscles involved in genitourinary control, used to control urinary flow. The transverse abdominis is not part of the pelvic floor muscles to control continence. Ab strengthening is not needed for continence training. That does not mean that continence cannot be trained. It is other muscles, not abdominals, that need the training. Train urinary continence by "holding" the stream. People sometimes tighten all the lower torso muscles when trying to figure out how to control the urinary constrictor muscles. However, bladder control does not require any tightening of the abdominal muscles.

Using them all
You don't have to know the names of the muscles to use them. You don't have to tighten them. Use them like other muscles to move your bones. Change your posture from arching to the back or sagging to the side during daily life and when you exercise. You'll have better posture, save your back, and get a workout by standing and moving properly.

Will Ab Revolution Exercises Hurt The Neck Or Back?

If doing anything from The Ab Revolution hurts, you are doing it wrong. Stop and check how to correct the movement. When using Ab Revolution exercises in Part II, you should feel effort, be sore from effort in the following days if you worked hard enough, but if it hurts, or causes new or more back pain, you ARE doing it wrong. If serious injury impedes any healthy movement, get evaluated to see what else is needed.

Many conventional abdominal exercises use spine and hip flexion. Chronic repeated forward bending is hard on your back and neck and does not train you how to stand and move with healthy spine and hip position when you get up off the floor or stop your "reps." The Ab Revolution trains abdominal strength and function without neck, back, or hip flexion. Both the component to stop back pain from hyperlordosis, Part I, and the exercise component, Part II, use your muscles to hold neutral spine the way you need for real life.

Don't tighten your joints or push them past their range. Don't bang your joints straight at the end of their range; use muscular control to avoid injury. Remember the purpose – healthier real life that is fun, and educates you to move in healthier ways, not grunting your way through an artificial exercise.

Used correctly, The Ab Revolution specifically trains you how to move in healthy positioning in daily life as well as during exercise, to prevent causes of neck and lower back pain.

Should You Work Your Abs Every Day or Every Other Day?

It is common to debate fiber type and fatigue to decide whether to exercise abdominal muscles daily or intermittently. Flurries of articles are written on which is correct.

What is missed is that, like your heart beating, you need your abdominal muscles working during all your daily movement. Doing crunches or any other ab exercise, then not using your abdominal muscles to control spine position the rest of the day; allowing painful injurious spine position, is missing the point of what abs are supposed to do. You are also missing an easy opportunity to burn calories, prevent back pain, and get a free all day workout.

You may exercise your abs and still have back pain, no matter whether you exercised every day or every few days. Don't miss the point that abdominal muscles need to be in use all the time, not by tightening, but used like any other skeletal muscles to move your bones into position. If you worked your abdominal muscles all the time to keep spine position healthy, you wouldn't need to go to a gym to do funny little crunches—not every day, nor every few days.

Why work out in order to use your abs, then allow hyperlordosis the rest of the day and undo your efforts? Stand, sit, lift, and reach well all the time and you will exercise your abdominal and core muscles without stopping your day to go "work out."

Is The Ab Revolution Researched As Effective?

The idea of research is to find what works and why, document it, test, and retest. The idea is not to take something you want to sell and try to prove it, or make it fit a model. The Ab Revolution method resulted over many years in the lab and with several thousands of students and participants over time, testing combinations of sports medicine rehabilitation techniques, healthy movement habits, and physical training methods, discarding what didn't work, retesting, and integrating what consistently resulted in improvements into real activities.

I started documenting my work developing this method in the 1970s from all students and patients who used it. When they used it as intended, results were high. I continued collecting data. I did more testing of results and printed the first training manual (typed actually, from hand printed notes) in 1982. I did university and military injury research in preventing back pain from running and carrying loads. Disease Non-Battle Injuries (DNBI) from exercising in the gym and doing PT is a huge military issue, grounding far more personnel than combat casualty. I ran several more studies on hyperlordosis, finding it is a major overlooked cause of lower back pain.

Back pain patients with hyperlordosis and facet pain usually learn to fix their pain from that problem during a single office visit, classroom instruction, or from reading and following written instructions, as in this book. They stop the pain from returning by continuing to use the healthier spine positioning.

I don't have a lot of time to publish my studies. I get direct critical evaluation and recommendations from reviewers and move to the next study to answer questions and question answers. Some of my more recent studies were presented at major sports medicine conferences and published in scientific peer review journals, resulting in a large amount of feedback which helped each subsequent study:

Bookspan, J. Comparison of Neutral Spine and Hamstring Stretch for Relief of Hyperlordotic Lumbar Pain *J. Medicine and Science in Sports and Exercise*, Volume 44:5 Supplement, 2012.

Bookspan, J. Comparison of Functional Lower Body Retraining and Conventional Strengthening in Knee Pain Resolution. *J. Medicine and Science in Sports and Exercise*, Volume 43:5 Supplement, 2011.

Bookspan, J. Hyperlordosis Retraining Method Relieves Spondylolisthesis Pain. *J. Medicine and Science in Sports and Exercise*, Volume 42:5 Supplement, 2010.

Bookspan, J. Hyperlordosis Retraining Method Relieves Lumbar Disc and Stenosis Pain - An Unexpected Finding. *J. Medicine and Science in Sports and Exercise*, Volume 41:5 Supplement, 2009

Bookspan, J. Identifying and Reversing Hyperlordosis as a Factor in Lower Back Pain. *J. Medicine and Science in Sports and Exercise*, Volume 39:5 Supplement, 2007.

Bookspan, J. Ab Revolution functional core retraining relieves low back pain more effectively than conventional physical therapy. *J. Medicine and Science in Sports and Exercise*, Volume 38:5 Supplement, 2006

Bookspan, J. Functional Core Retraining Superior To Conventional And Pilates Core Training In Remediating Low Back Pain. *J. Medicine and Science in Sports and Exercise*, Volume 37:5, 2005.

Work is ongoing to identify injurious movement, to create injury-preventing technique, and develop effective training methods that are healthful for real-world activities.

Why Is This Method Called a Revolution?

The Ab Revolution is a researched sports medicine modality. It was given its non-medical sounding name when laboratory research showed that standard core exercises and explanation of core function were the reverse of what really happens. The method became a revolution in core training – a change in thinking of how core muscles work and what they do, in using them in real life, and understanding their relation to a common form of back pain.

Abdominal exercise is often thought of as stopping real life to lie on the floor, or use machines, or hunch and bend forward in motions that are not the way you move in real life, but may make your neck hurt and often your back too. The assumption for these exercises is that strengthening the muscles automatically does something to change the lower back or posture. It does not work that way. Strengthening alone does not automatically change posture, prevent the cause of back pain, or teach how you use your muscles in real activities. Many people with strong muscles and tight abs have poor posture, injurious spinal positioning, and persistent back pain.

The Ab Revolution shows how to use abdominal and core muscles to change spine position to neutral, then apply the healthy new position to all you do during daily life and exercise. This simple technique is key in how using muscles (not merely having them) keeps injurious forces off your back during daily activities. Conventional ab exercises don't transfer these specific positioning skills to real life. The very thing we regard as exercise advice, "do sets and reps (however many) of crunches," is one of the problems because it separates exercise from how to use muscles to move in healthy ways in real life. Ab exercise has become hugely popularized as something you specially "do" then never transfer the specific function that you need your abs to do— hold your spine in neutral. Abdominal and core exercise is used in many back pain rehabilitation programs, but pain often returns because neutral spine position or any needed change in posture or function or healthy movement skills does not happen automatically from doing bent forward abdominal exercises or strengthening.

Using abdominal muscles is not "tightening" them. You cannot move or breathe properly that way, and tight muscles are a factor in headaches, poor posture, and back pain. Tightening does not move your spine out of unhealthful position into neutral spine. The Ab Revolution does.

The Ab Revolution builds abdominal and core muscles and their best use, without crunches or forward bending. It challenges the muscles to hold neutral spine to strengthen them functionally while specifically training you to keep neutral spine during daily life. Conventional forward bending does not teach to use your body the way you need for real life once you get off the floor. In other words, it is not functional. Moreover, crunches, leg lifts, and other forward bending positions can be counterproductive after a day of bending forward over a desk, steering wheel, and everything else.

The Ab Revolution is a change in understanding about abs and their function. It gives information of what abs really do, what they don't do, and how to consciously use your abs to position your spine and hip for all your activities. It teaches specific skills to make your life better. The exercises strengthen your abdominal muscles, together with your back, arms, shoulders, and legs, and teach you how your muscles need to work together in your real life.

By following the techniques in this book, you get exercise without going to a gym. You strengthen abdominal muscles without forward bending. You strengthen your body as a whole while getting abdominal exercise. You burn calories. You stop one of the main injurious postures that creates back pain. You exercise your brain.

It's a sea change. It's a transformation. It's a paradigm shift. Those didn't make a good name for this method. It's a revolution.

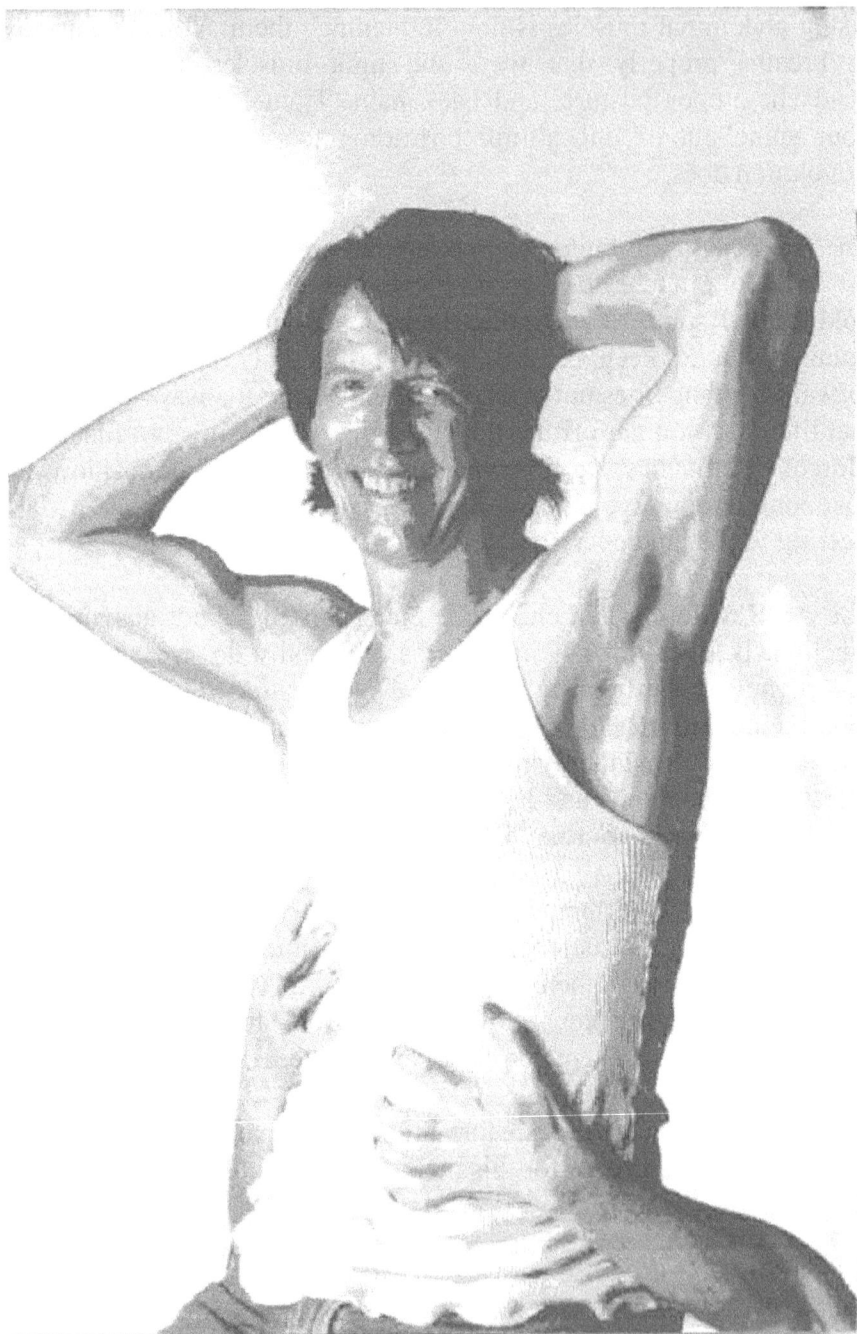

Get fun and benefit with this method.

What Instructors and Trainers Say About The Ab Revolution

"You have eliminated my longstanding back pain. Thank you for constantly discrediting the myths that are so-often forced upon us."
—*Audrey Tannenbaum, M.Ed., A.T.C., C.S.C.S., Athletic Trainer and Maccabean Games Triathlon Gold Medalist*

"This class dispelled many myths about abs. I've learned many exercises to bring to my group fitness classes."
—*Jack Sannino, Group exercise instructor*

"The Ab Revolution is a whole new way of life and a better way of doing abs. I have already reduced my own back pain. Great new method."
—*Mary Ann Rahman, Aerobics teacher*

"I like this method. It is energetic, fun, & makes excellent functional sense. I've learned how to use my abs for every day, all day."
—*Tracy Selekman, National Strength & Conditioning Association Certified Personal Trainer*

"I've incorporated so much of your good advice into my yoga classes. I end each class with a period of lying on the floor and using the ab muscles to keep the lumber spine in place while moving the arms - a variation of the *Isometric Abs* exercise. Many students had previously bent knees for this. After the lumbar work, I find that almost all have straight, extended legs in complete relaxation. They notice that they are more comfortable afterward and able to sit and stand straighter. Hooooooray!!"
—*Peggy Santamaria, AFEM Director of Developmental Ability*

What Black Belt Martial Artists Say About The Ab Revolution

"This was a tremendously enlightening approach to core training. It will allow me to continue martial arts for many years. "
   —*Andrew Seigel, 3rd Degree Black Belt Modern Bujitsu*

"The Ab Revolution already helped my back pain. I use it in all my martial arts training to change to correct technique. This technique will relieve a lot of pain from incorrectly performing our exercises."
   — *Richard Bole, PHG, PA 2nd Degree Black Belt*

"Excellent knowledge and workout on abs. The Ab Revolution already helped my back pain. I will have less trouble with my lower back during training now at age 62. Valuable information that I can pass on to our students."
   —*Eb Molesch, 7th Degree Black Belt*

"No more crunches and a better understanding of physiology. Check this out! "
   —*Jacqueline Prats, 2nd Degree Black Belt Tang Soo Do, Jiu Jitsu, Aikido*

"The workshop made me more cognizant of myths and better training. Of all the fitness people I've spoken to over the years, you put the correct focus on how to do it correctly and why. I hope we can attend another of your seminars. The book is a must-read."
   —Denise Molesch. 4th Degree Black Belt Tae Kwon Do

What Medical Doctors Say About The Ab Revolution

"Well, Jolie Bookspan has done it again! An expert at debunking "scientific" bunk, she has developed an extremely effective method that can be used in every day life for the thousands (millions?) who have chronic lumbosacral pain. Freeing the "crunchers" from the boredom of useless exercise programs that are quickly abandoned, the program is simple, sensible, and highly effective. Highly recommended."
> —*Ernest Campbell, M.D., FACS, President of the Medical Staff, Chairman of the Department of Surgery, Board of Directors, Brookwood Medical Center*

"I've given *The Ab Revolution* to my physical therapists and trainers to use. You have condensed things to a very workable format."
> —*Stanley A. Herring M.D., FACSM, Puget Sound Sports & Spine Physicians, Former President of the North American Spine Society*

"I have learned how to teach patients to treat their back pain. Superb instructor."
> —*Fabrice Czarnecki, M.D., Family and Travel Medicine, Johns Hopkins*

"It's about time someone looked at the real science behind the movements, not mindlessly putting people through the exercises."
> —*Thomas M. Bozzuto, D.O., Medical Director Baptist Health System Wound Care Center*

"This is a method that everyone interested in good health and muscle tone should learn, especially trainers."
  —*J. Tom Millington, M.D., Medical Director, St. John's Pleasant Valley Hospital*

"Whenever I have a question on rehab, or want practical advice on fitness training or musculoskeletal complaints, I turn to my friend and colleague, Dr. Jolie Bookspan. I trust her for good sense and her solid background in exercise physiology."
  —*David Hsu, M.D., Ph.D., Neurology, Stanford Medical Center*

"If I were to say something sage about exercise, I am afraid that others will die laughing since my aversion to exercise is well known. I always wanted to have you as my personal trainer because you are the only person in the world who might get me to think otherwise about exercise."
  —*Caroline Fife, M.D., Associate Professor, Department of Anesthesiology, University of Texas Health Science Center, Houston. Chief Consultant, CHeCS Training Program Krug Life Sciences NASA*

"Dr. Bookspan, the brightest light in popular sports medicine, cuts through the myths and falsehoods about abs."
  —*Kelly Hill, M.D., FACSM, Green Beret Lt. Colonel, SWAT Team Commander*

More Resources by Jolie Bookspan
http://drbookspan.com/

Health & Fitness in Plain English
Third edition. How To Be Healthy Happy and Fit for the Rest of Your Life. Thirty-one fun chapters, exercise, nutrition, health of bone, blood, heart, joints, funny facts, preventive medicine, and other topics for healthier life. 376 pages, illustrated.

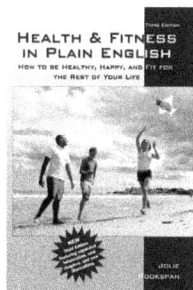

Healthy Martial Arts
Wealth of Innovative training for *all* athletes. Train body and mind, reduce injury. 232 pages. Over 200 photos. Beautiful print edition and full color e-Book. Winner of the Eastern USA International Black Belt Hall of Fame Reader's Choice Award.

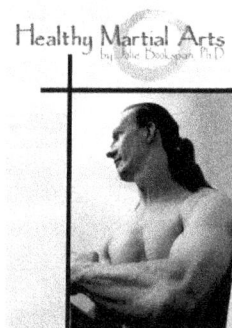

Fix Your Own Pain
Without Drugs or Surgery
Back pain, neck pain, shoulder, knee, foot, ankle and hip pain, fasciitis, disc pain, sciatica, lordosis, flat feet, carpal tunnel, "everything hurts" with fun stories from real patients.

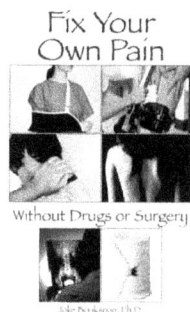

Stretching Smarter, Stretching Healthier. Fun, easy to read, immediately helpful changes. 106 pages. Over 200 humorous illustrations guide you step-by-step.

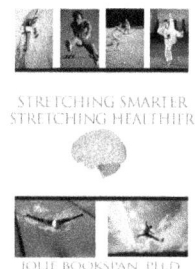

Diving Physiology in Plain English
The book for every scuba diver, novice to instructor, and their health providers. Clear information to understand (not memorize) physiology and medicine, and apply to safer decompression, thermal, equipment, gas mixing, fitness to dive, nutrition, rescue, injuries, and to demystify the many claims and counterclaims in diving. Complex topics translated into understanding. Fun stories and illustrated glossary. 6th printing revised with new blue cover. 246 pages, illustrated.

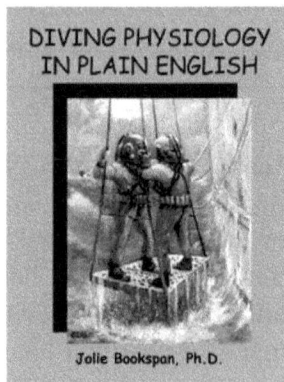
DIVING PHYSIOLOGY IN PLAIN ENGLISH
Jolie Bookspan, Ph.D.

Diving and Hyperbaric Medicine Review For Physicians
Extensive compendium of information to work in hyperbaric medicine and take the board exam. Includes diving medicine, physiology, diving and hyperbaric history, practice, physics, and clinical hyperbaric treatment of wound healing, diving and non-diving conditions. Reviews entire field, in quick, bulleted points. Includes sample ABPM board exam questions on each topic with answers. 226 pages.

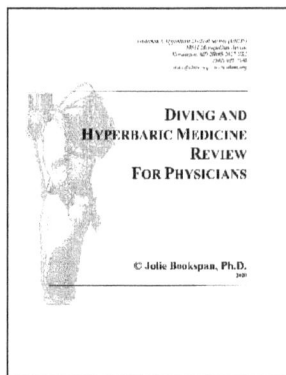
DIVING AND HYPERBARIC MEDICINE REVIEW FOR PHYSICIANS
© Jolie Bookspan, Ph.D.

Hyperbaric Medical Review For Certified Hyperbaric Technologist (CHT) and Certified Hyperbaric Registered Nurse (CHRN)
Required knowledge for chamber nurses and technicians to work in the field & take board exams. Includes the TCom module and sample board exam questions and answers. 190 pages.

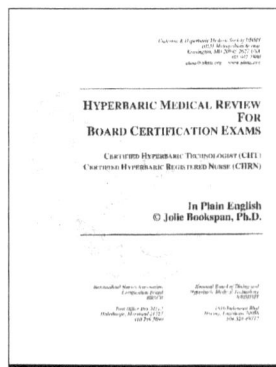
HYPERBARIC MEDICAL REVIEW FOR BOARD CERTIFICATION EXAMS
Certified Hyperbaric Technologist (CHT) Certified Hyperbaric Registered Nurse (CHRN)
In Plain English
© Jolie Bookspan, Ph.D.

Credits

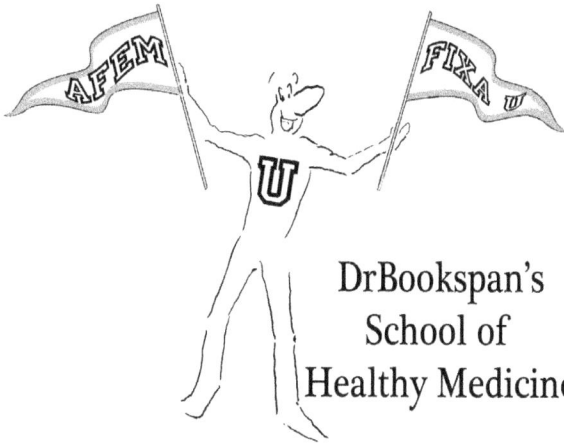

DrBookspan's
School of
Healthy Medicine

Backman!™ drawings for teaching healthy movement. Concept, prototype, and most drawings by Jolie Bookspan. Model by Todd Sargood.

Academy logo by Alessandro Schiavone, Ravenna Italy.

Fixa U logo and Neck and Back Pain Sports Medicine logos © Jolie Bookspan.

Some images ©2006 JupiterImages, Clipart.com, by subscription.

Helpful edits, Thomas H. Kohn, Esq.

Author photos by Robert Troia.

Photo of cover model Paul Plevakas by Vision 13 Photography.

Photo models for drills are Dr. Bookspan's dedicated hard-working students. If you see yourself and are not mentioned here, get in touch:

Shelly Anthony	Elsa Leung
Regina Basile	Rhonda McJeff
Nahy Milad Bassil	Stacia Mellbourne
Cynthia Brown	Travis Mesman
Emily Canon	Jim Passio
Louis Costa	Sara Rathfon
Dr. Martin Dembitzer	Danielle Tobin
Angela and Andrea Fleegle	Paul J and son James

About the Author

Dr. Bookspan knows abs. Military scientist, 4th degree black belt, undefeated in the ring as a Muay Thai fighter, and research physiologist studying survival in extremes from undersea to mountain top to outer space, an interest that began as a child sitting barefoot in the snow watching her grandfather go ice swimming every day. As a scientist, she carried gear up and down the mountains and deserts of India, Nepal, Asia, and Northern Africa; swam to work in an underwater laboratory; was advisor to The Discovery Channel and police and military training departments; and professor of anatomy at a college in the mountains of Mexico where the entrance exam was getting up there without a nosebleed. Left paralyzed after breaking her back, neck, and most of everything else in an accident, she rehabbed using her own methods, started over as a white belt until earning the black belt a second time. Inducted, with husband Paul, to the International Black Belt Hall of Fame Martial Arts Association, Martial Arts Man and Women of the Year 2004, and Instructors of the Year 2009. Harvard medical school clinicians named her, "The St. Jude of the Joints."

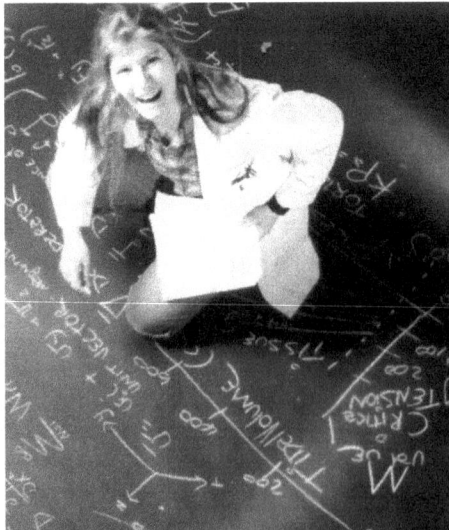

www.ingramcontent.com/pod-product-compliance
Lightning Source LLC
Chambersburg PA
CBHW072132020426
42334CB00018B/1766